Lang
Ward

MW01093035

Essential Evidence-based Data for
Common Clinical Encounters

Anil Patel, MD

Department of Family Medicine
University of Pittsburgh Medical Center
Pittsburgh, Pennsylvania

McGraw-Hill
Medical Publishing Division

New York Chicago San Francisco Lisbon London
Madrid Mexico City Milan New Delhi San Juan Seoul
Singapore Sydney Toronto

Lange Instant Access: Wards

Essential Evidence-based Data for Common Clinical Encounters

Copyright © 2006 by The McGraw-Hill Companies, Inc. All rights reserved. Printed in the United States of America. Except as permitted under the United States Copyright Act of 1976, no part of this publication may be reproduced or distributed in any form or by any means, or stored in a data base or retrieval system, without the prior written permission of the publisher.

1 2 3 4 5 6 7 8 9 0 DOC/DOC 0 9 8 7 6

ISBN 0-07-147165-0

Notice

Medicine is an ever-changing science. As new research and clinical experience broaden our knowledge, changes in treatment and drug therapy are required. The authors and the publisher of this work have checked with sources believed to be reliable in their efforts to provide information that is complete and generally in accord with the standards accepted at the time of publication. However, in view of the possibility of human error or changes in medical sciences, neither the authors nor the publisher nor any other party who has been involved in the preparation or publication of this work warrants that the information contained herein is in every respect accurate or complete, and they disclaim all responsibility for any errors or omissions or for the results obtained from use of the information contained in this work. Readers are encouraged to confirm the information contained herein with other sources. For example and in particular, readers are advised to check the product information sheet included in the package of each drug they plan to administer to be certain that the information contained in this work is accurate and that changes have not been made in the recommended dose or in the contraindications for administration. This recommendation is of particular importance in connection with new or infrequently used drugs.

This book was set in Palatino by International Typesetting and Composition.
The editors were Jim Shanahan and Maya Barahona.
The production supervisor was Sherri Souffrance.
Project management was provided by International Typesetting and Composition.
The cover designer was Mary McKeon.
RR Donnelley was printer and binder.
This book is printed on acid-free paper.

Contents

Contributors

Beena Ahmad, MD
Internal Medicine, PGY III
UPMC, Pittsburgh, Pennsylvania

Robert Barnabei, MD
Inpatient Director and Clinical Instructor, Family Medicine
UPMC, Pittsburgh, Pennsylvania

Daphne Bicket, MD
Associate Clinical Instructor, Family Medicine
UPMC, Pittsburgh, Pennsylvania

Veena Dhar, MD
Clinical Instructor, Family Medicine,
UPMC, Pittsburgh, Pennsylvania

David Garzarelli, MD
Associate Program Director & Clinical Assistant Professor,
    Family Medicine
UPMC, Pittsburgh, Pennsylvania

Indira Jevaji, MD
Clinical Assistant Professor, Family Medicine
UPMC, Pittsburgh, Pennsylvania

Madhusudan Menon, MD
Associate Program Director and Inpatient Director,
    Internal Medicine
UPMC, Pittsburgh, Pennsylvania

Gustavo Ortiz, MD
Neurology, PGY IV, Jackson Memorial Hospital
University of Miami, Miami, Florida

Anil M. Patel, MD
Family Medicine Resident (PGY—III)
University of Pittsburgh Medical Center (UPMC)
Pittsburgh, Pennsylvania

Thomas Powell, MD
Clinical Instructor, Department of Nephrology
UPMC, Pittsburgh, Pennsylvania

Renato Samala, MD
Internal Medicine, PGY III
UPMC, Pittsburgh, Pennsylvania

Joseph Secosky, MD
Clinical Instructor, Department of Cardiology
UPMC, Pittsburgh, Pennsylvania

Shripal Shrishrimal, MD
Internal Medicine, PGY III
UPMC, Pittsburgh, Pennsylvania

Phoebe Tobiano, MD
Family Medicine, PGY III, Chief Resident
UPMC, Pittsburgh, Pennsylvania

Preface

This book presents essential facts and data that are inherently part of the patient care encounters faced by new clinicians. It was written to be used independently, but it can also be used as a companion to the standard handbooks of clinical medicine, many of which focus on step-by-step guidance to the clinical methods of diagnosis and treatment. *Lange Instant Access: Wards* presents the high-yield facts and data that underlie patient presentations and diseases and clinical interventions. The abbreviated length was chosen so as to make the information in the book as quickly retrievable as possible.

Lange Instant Access: Wards was written for third and fourth year medical students and interns.

It includes evidence-based information, essential for today's learning, and covers multiple topics in both primary care and the medical subspecialties. The content of each chapter was based on the most commonly asked questions among medical students and residents. All the materials were acquired from respected references in the medical literature and are cited throughout. The unique aspect of this book is its formatting. A table format was chosen to promote easy readability and recall and facilitate quick reference.

This book is a product of two years of hard work, which was reviewed by some of the most recognized and respected physicians in Family Medicine and Internal Medicine. We were struck by the prepublication reviews from medical students, interns, and residents in the specialties of Primary Care, including:

- "Well organized and easy to find information."
- "Concise and does not include extraneous material."
- "All major topics in the specialties are covered."
- "Nice concise reference of high-yield facts and topics."
- "I wish this book was available when I was in my 3rd year."

This book will be helpful to all in their journey to becoming a great physician.

Acknowledgments

I would like to thank my parents for their support. I would also like all the editors and contributors for their time and work devoted to this book. Also, I would like to thank James Shanahan, Maya Barahona, and Gita Raman for working very closely with me in making *Lange Instant Access: Wards* a reality.

00
Guide Tables

TABLE 00–1: Commonly Used Symbols	
$\circ \rightarrow$ hour	$♀ \rightarrow$ female
$\psi \rightarrow$ psychiatric/psychiatry	$♂ \rightarrow$ male
$\Theta \rightarrow$ no or negative	$\uparrow \rightarrow$ increase/up/greater/high
$\rightarrow$ no or negative	$\downarrow \rightarrow$ decrease/down/less/low
$\Delta \rightarrow$ change	$\leftrightarrow \rightarrow$ no change
$\beta \rightarrow$ beta	
$\begin{array}{cc|c} Na & Cl & BUN \\ \hline K & HCO_3 & Creatinine \end{array}$ Glucose	$\begin{matrix} \text{Hemoglobin} \\ \text{WBC} \diagdown \diagup \text{Platelets} \quad \text{PT} \diagup \diagdown \text{PTT} \\ \text{Hematocrit} \qquad \diagup \text{INR} \diagdown \end{matrix}$
Calcium/magnesium/PO_4	ABG = pH/$PaCO_2$/PaO_2/ HCO_3/oxygen sat/base deficit

TABLE 00–2: Conversions

Weight	Volume	Distance	Temperature
1 lb = 0.453 kg	1 fluid oz = 30 mL	1 cm = 0.394 in.	$F = (1.8)C + 32$
1 kg = 2.216 lb	1 Tsp = 5 mL	1 m = 3.28 ft	$C = (F - 32)/(1.8)$
1 lb = 16 oz	1 Tbs = 15 mL	1 km = 0.621 mi	
1 oz = 28.35 g	1 Tbs = 3 Tsp	**Other**	
1 grain = 65 mg	1 fl dram = 4 mL	$Mmol/L = [mg/dL \times 10]/mol\ wt$	
	1 gal = 3.79 L	$meq/L = mmol/L \times valence$	
Tbs =	1 mg = 1000 μg		
	1 gal = 128 oz		

Ideal body weight (IBW) = for male → 106 lb for 5 ft and 6 lb for each inch above 5 ft for female → 100 lb for 5 ft and 5 lb for each inch above 5 ft

Body mass index (BMI) = wt (lb)/ht (in.)$^2 \times 704.5$ or wt (kg)/ ht (m)^2

Abbreviations: Tbs, tablespoon; Tsp, teaspoon.

TABLE 00–3: Temperature Conversion					
°F	95	96	97	98	98.6	99
°C	35	35.6	36.1	36.7	37	37.2
°F	101	102	103	104	105	106
°C	38.3	38.9	39.4	40	40.6	41.1

TABLE 00–4: Dangerous Abbreviations	
Do Not Use	**Use**
QD/qd	Daily
QOD	Every other day
MS, MSO_4, $MgSO_4$	Magnesium sulfate or morphine sulfate
U or u	Unit(s)
IU	International Unit(s)
Trailing zero: 1.0	1
Lack of leading zero: .1	0.1
µg	Microgram
SQ or SC	Sub Q
CC or Cc	mL or ML
Os	Left
Od	Right
Ou	Both

1
Allergy & Immunology

TABLE 1–1: Rash (Allergic, Eczema, Contact Dermatitis, Pruritus)

→ R/O anaphylactic RXN and drug reaction

→ Benadryl 50 mg PO/IV/IM q4-6h (caution in elderly, it may cause delirium) or

→ Atarax 50–100 mg PO/IM q4-6h

→ Cimetidine 400 mg PO q4-6 with H_1 blocker

→ Eucerin lotion/Eucerin plus lotion: used for xerosis (dry skin)

→ Pepcid 20 mg PO bid

→ Steroid topical

1. **Low potency**

   • Hydrocortisone acetate (Cortaid) 0.5% C L O, 1% C F O bid–qid

   • Hydrocortisone 0.25% C L, 0.5%, 1%, 2.5%, C L O S, 2% L bid–qid

   • Desonide 0.05% C L O bid–tid

2. **Medium potency**

   • Mometasone furoate (Elocon) C L O 0.1% daily

   • Triamcinolone (Aristocort) 0.025%, 0.1% C L O bid–tid

   • Flurandrenolide (Cordran) 0.025% C O, 0.05% C L O bid–qid

TABLE 1–1 (Continued)

3. High potency

- Triamcinolone acetonide (Kenalog, Aristocort) 0.5% C bid–tid

- Amcinonide (Cyclocort) 0.05% C L O daily–tid

4. Super high potency

- Betamethasone diproprionate (Diprolene) 0.05% C G L O daily–bid

Abbreviations: C, cream; F, foam; G, gel; L, lotion; O, ointment; S, solution.

TABLE 1–2: Acute Allergic Reaction

Meds	Dose (Adult)	Dose (Pediatric)
Diphenhydramine (Benadryl)	25–50 mg PO/IM/IV	1–2 mg/kg PO
Loratadine (Claritin)	10 mg PO	5 mg PO
Cetirizine (Zyrtec)	5–10 mg PO	2.5–5.0 mg PO
Prednisone	40–60 mg PO	1–2 mg/kg PO
A. Mild–Moderate Anaphylaxis		
Epinephrine 1/1000 (1 mg/1 mL)	Epi-Pen 0.3 mg IM	Epi-Pen Jr. 0.15 mg IM
Diphenhydramine (Benadryl)	25–50 mg PO, IM, IV	1–2 mg/kg PO, IM, IV
Ranitidine (Zantac)	50 mg IV	1–1.5 mg IV
Cimetidine (Tagamet)	300 mg IV	5 mg/kg IV
Prednisone	40–60 mg PO	1–2 mg/kg PO
Methylprednisolone (Medrol)	125 mg IV/IM	1–2 mg/kg IV/IM

TABLE 1–2 (Continued)		
B. Severe Anaphylaxis (Treat as Above Plus Add the Following)		
• **Epinephrine**		
1/10,000 (1 mg/10 mL)	0.005 mg/kg (0.05 mL/kg IV in 10 mL NS) give over 5 min	0.01 mg/kg (0.1mL/ kg IV in 10 mL NS) give over 5 min
1/100,000 (1 mg/100 mL)	0.75–1.5 mg/kg IV slowly	

Source: Reproduced with permission from Gavalas M, Sadana A, Metcalf S. Guidelines for the managements of anaphylaxis in emergency department. *J Accid Emerg med* 1998;15:96–98.

TABLE 1–3: Blood Transfusion Reaction

A. Febrile nonhemolytic transfusion reaction

Si/Sx: fever, chills, mild dyspnea within 1–6 h after transfusion

Labs: R/O acute hemolytic transfusion reaction, see below for labs

Management

- Stop the transfusion

- Administer acetaminophen 650 mg 1 tab PO

- If severe chills and rigor

  A. Meperidine 50–100 mg PO q2-4h or IM, Sub Q, 50–75 mg every 3–4 h prn

(If CrCl < 10 mL/min: administer 50% of normal dose)

  ■ Elderly: 50 mg PO q4h prn or IM: 25 mg q4h

  ■ Renal impairment: CrCl → 10–50 mL/min: give 75% of normal dose

B. Acute hemolytic transfusion reaction

Si/Sx: triad—fever, flank pain, and red urine; chills

(If DIC → patient may be oozing from puncture sites)

- Stop the transfusion but leave IV access

Labs

- Inform blood bank

- Send the current PRBC bag back to blood bank for re-type and cross

TABLE 1–3 (Continued)
• Order transfusion reaction panel
• From other arm: check for a direct Coombs test and for plasma free Hb
• Check for urine for Hb testing (Urine R&M)
• Check with blood bank on their protocol for transfusion reaction
Management
• Check for clerical error
• Transfuse NS (do not use Ringers/Dextrose) at 100–200 mL/h
• Vigorous supportive care is essential
• Cautious heparinization (10 units/kg/h) for 12–24 h to prevent DIC
• Dopamine can be used as vasopressor
• Hyperkalemia is likely: cardiac monitoring and hemodialysis may be required
• Alkalinization in marked hemoglobinuria is controversial
C. Anaphylactic transfusion reactions
Si/Sx: rapid onset of shock, hypotension, angioedema, respiratory distress, laryngeal edema, and bronchospasm
Labs
• See acute hemolytic transfusion reaction

TABLE 1–3 (Continued)

Management

- Stop the transfusion

- Airway maintenance and oxygenation

- Epinephrine 0.3 mL of 1:1000 solution IM

- Prepare IV epinephrine drip

- Maintain volume with IV NS

- Vasopressors (Dopamine) if needed

D. Delayed hemolytic transfusion reaction (seen 2–10 days after transfusion)

Si/Sx: slight fever, falling HCT

Labs

- Mild ↑ in serum unconjugated bilirubin, spherocytosis on blood smear

Management

- No treatment is required in the absence of brisk hemolysis; however, offending antigen need to be identified for future transfusion

TABLE 1–4: Allergic Conjunctivitis

- 1st line → Naphcon 1–2 drops qid (do not use >3 weeks) or

    → Ocuhist 1–2 drops qid (do not use >3 weeks)

    → Visine AC 1–2 drops qid (do not use >3 weeks)

- 2nd line → Patanol 1–2 drops bid or

    → Acular 1–2 drops qid

- 3rd line → use in conjunction with 1st and 2nd line treatment as above

    → Alomide 1–2 drops qid or

    → Opticrom 1–2 drops qid or

    → Crolom 1–2 drops qid

TABLE 1–5: Acute Urticaria and Angioedema

History is essential in determining the etiology

Labs	
• CBC with Diff	• ESR
• LFT	• UA
• Skin testing for allergens	• ?ANA
• ? TSH	• ?Hepatitis panel

Management
1. Avoid specific allergen
2. Oral H_1 antagonist (see Table 1–2)
3. Add H_2 antagonist in resistant cases
4. If anaphylaxis (see anaphylactic reaction management in this chapter)
? means this test may be ordered but clinical correlation required

TABLE 1–6: Chronic Urticaria

History is essential in determining the etiology

Labs

• CBC with Diff	• ESR
• LFT	• UA
• Skin testing for allergens	• ANA
• TSH	• Hepatitis panel
• Thyroid microsomal antibodies	• Thyroglobulin antibodies
• C1q	• C2
• C4	• C1 esterase inhibitor

• Eosinophilia suggests drug, food, or parasitic causes

• ANA and ESR should be performed in patient with connective tissue dz. symptoms

• Biopsy of hives which last longer than 36 h (to rule out urticarial vasculitis)

Management for Urticaria

1. Avoid specific allergen

2. 2nd Generation H_1 antihistamines: cetirizine (Zyrtec), loratadine (Claritin), fexofenadine higher than suggested doses may be required

3. Add H_2 antagonist for adequate control

4. Hydroxyzine or doxepin can be taken at night due to its sedating effect

TABLE 1–6 (Continued)

5. Systemic steroids can be useful for temporary relief

6. STOP cigarette, cosmetics, toiletries, cleaning solution, aerosol, antacid, laxative

7. Leukotrine receptor antagonists (zafirlukast and monte-lukast can be useful in combination with H_2)

8. Cyclosporine 20 mg daily can be useful in patient who responds poorly to antihistamines

Management for Angioedema

1. ABCs

2. Stanozolol 4 mg q4h

3. Antihistamines and corticosteroids are also useful

4. Airway compromise or vasomotor instability, patient should immediately receive epinephrine. Administer epinephrine (1:1000) 0.3–0.5 mL IM q15-20min

TABLE 1–7: Medications in Urticaria		
Name	**Tablet Form**	**Liquid Form**
H_1 Antagonist (Sedating)		
Diphenhydramine	25–50 mg bid–qid	Elixir: 12.5 mg/5 mL
		Syrup: 6.25 mg/5 mL
Hydroxyzine (Atarax)	10–50 mg qid	10 mg/5 mL
		Susp: 25 mg/5 mL
Cyproheptadine (Periactin)	4–8 mg qid	2 mg/5 mL
H_1 Antagonist (Non-sedating)		
Fexofenadine (Allegra)	180 mg daily–bid	
Cetirizine (Zyrtec)	10 mg daily–bid	5 mg/5 mL
Desloratadine (Clarinex)	5–10 mg daily	
Loratadine (Claritin)	10–20 mg daily–bid	5 mg/5 mL
H_2 Antagonist		
Cimetidine (Tagamet)	400–800 mg bid	300 mg/5 mL
Famotidine (Pepcid)	20–40 mg	40 mg/5 mL
Ranitidine (Zantac)	150–300 mg bid	75 mg/5 mL

TABLE 1–7 (Continued)		
H$_1$ and H$_2$ Receptor Antagonist		
Doxepin (Sinequan)	10–50 mg qid	10 mg/mL
Corticosteroids		
Methylprednisolone (Medrol)	16 mg every other day with gradual taper	
Prednisone	20 mg every other day with gradual taper	5 mg/mL
Leukotriene Antagonist		
Zafirlukast (Accolate)	20 mg bid	
Montelukast (Singulair)	10 mg daily	
Immunotherapy		
Cyclosporine	2–3 mg/kg starting then 4–6 mg/kg	100 mg/mL
Methotrexate	2.5 mg bid for 3 days of the week	25 mg/mL
	5 mg bid for 3 days of the week	
Epinephrine		
Ana-Guard (1:1000)	0.3 mL/dose Sub Q	
Epi-Pen Jr. (1:2000)	<12 years (0.15 mg/dose)	
Epi-Pen (1:1000)	0.3 mg/dose	

2
Cardiology

TABLE 2–1: Useful Formulas

- A-a gradient (5–15 on room air) = $[(713 \times FiO_2) - (PaCO_2/0.8)] - PaO_2$

- Cardiac output (CO) = $HR \times SV$ (4–6 L/min)

- Cardiac index (CI) = $CO \times BSA$ (2.5–3.5 L/min/m^2)

- Ejection fraction (>55%) = (SV × 100/end diastolic volume)

- Mean arterial pressure (70–100) = $[(2 \times \text{diastolic BP}) + (\text{systolic BP})/3]$

- Mean arterial pressure (70–100) = diastolic BP + ($1/3 \times$ pulse pressure)

- Pulse pressure = systolic BP – diastolic BP

- Max predicted HRT = 220 – age

- SVR = 80(MAP – CVP)/CO

- QTc (corrected QT) = QT interval/square root of RR interval (millisecond)

TABLE 2–2: ECG Reading[a]

Intervals and Lead Areas

• One small box = 0.04 s or 1 mm	• Anteroseptal wall → V_1 and V_2
• One large box = 0.2 s or 5 mm	• Anterior wall → V_3 and V_4
• P wave → <0.11 s	• Anterolateral wall → V_5 and V_6
• P-R interval → 0.12–0.2 s	• High lateral → I and aVL
• QRS complex → <0.07–0.10 s	• Inferior wall → leads II, III, and AVF
• QTc interval → 0.33–0.47 s	• Lateral leads → I, AVL, V_5, and V_6

• QTc (corrected QT interval) = QT interval/square root of RR interval (millisecond)

A. Rate

• Count # large boxes between R-R and divide 300 by the number of boxes

• Count # large boxes between R-R in 10 seconds multiplied by 6

• Per big boxes: 300-150-100-75-60

(continued)

TABLE 2–2 (Continued)			
B. Rhythm			
P wave followed by QRS → sinus	Regular	<60 bpm	Sinus bradycardia
		60–100 bpm	Normal sinus rhythm
		>100 bpm	Sinus tachycardia
	Irregular	Sinus arrhythmia	
No p waves	Irregularly irregular	Atrial fib	
	Regular	Slow/normal	Junctional/ idioventricular rhythm
		Rapid	SVT/A flutter
		Wide complex	Monomorphic V-Tech
			Polymorphic torsades de pointes

TABLE 2–2 (Continued)				
PR interval (0.12–0.2 s)	1st degree AV block	Constant prolonged PR interval >0.2 (200 ms)	
	2nd degree AV block	Gradual PR prolongation with sudden drop	Mobitz type I Wenckebach
		Constant PR (not prolonged) with sudden drop	Mobitz type II
	3rd degree AV block	QRS doesn't follow P P-P interval constant R-R interval constant	

C. Axis			
Lead I	Lead AVF	Lead II[b]	Axis
(+)[c]	(+)	(+)	Normal
(+)	(−)[d]	(−)	Left
(−)	(+)	(+)	Right
(−)	(−)	(−)	Right or indeterminate if AVR+

(continued)

TABLE 2–2 (Continued)	
D. QRS Duration	
<0.10 s	Normal
0.10–0.12 s	Incomplete BBB or LAFB/LPFB
	LAFB (left anterior fascicular block) = LAD + Q_1S_3
	LPFB (left posterior fascicular block) = RAD + Q_3S_1
>0.12 s	Complete RBBB (RSR' in V_1)
	LBBB; nonspecific intraventricular conduction delay (qr or q)
	Bifascicular block = RBBB + LAFB
E. Hypertrophies	

RAE	Lead II P wave > 2.5 mm (aka P-pulmonale)	
LAE	V_1 P wave negative deflection > 1 block wide and > 1 block deep (aka P-mitrale)	
LVH	1. R wave in aVL > 12 mm 2. (S wave in V_1 or V_2 whichever is larger) + (R wave in V_5 or V_6 whichever is larger) ≥ 35 mm	
RVH	1. R > S in V_1 2. R decreases from V_1 to V_6	

TABLE 2–2 (Continued)	
F. Prolonged QTc Etiologies (See Table 2–1)	
Medications	**Miscellaneous Medications**
Antibiotics	Phenylamine
Azithromycin, erythromycin, clarithromycin	Cisapride
Telithromycin	Domperidone
Levofloxacin, moxifloxacin, gatifloxacin	Droperidol
Sparfloxacin	Probucol
Pentamidine	Cocaine
Spiramycin, chloroquine, halofantrine, mefloquine	Terodiline
Antihistamines	Papaverine
Astemizole	Chloral hydrate
Terfenadine	Arsenic
Antiarrhythmics	Cesium chloride
Amiodarone	Levomethadyl
Disopyramide	**Metabolic etiology**
Dofetilide, sematilide, ibutilide, bepridil, mibefradil	Hypokalemia
Procainamide/ N-acetylprocainamide	Hypomagnesemia

(continued)

TABLE 2–2 (Continued)	
Quinidine	Hypocalcemia
Sotalol	Hypothyroidism
Psychotropics	Starvation
Butorphanol	**Miscellaneous**
Haloperidol	Idiopathic
Methadone (high dose)	Mitral valve prolapse
Phenothiazines	Myocardial ischemia/ infarction
Risperidone	HIV
SSRI	Hypothermia
TCA	Connective tissue disease
Thioridazine	Jervell–Lange–Nielsen and Romano–Ward syndrome

TABLE 2–2 (Continued)

G. Miscellaneous

- COPD pattern: precordial leads R/S ratio <1

- Chronic lung disease: poor R wave progression, P-pulmonale, MAT (multifocal atrial tachycardia)

- T wave flattening: ischemia, hypokalemia, or nonspecific

- U wave: hypokalemia, ischemia

- QT shortening: hypercalcemia

- QT prolongation: hypocalcemia, other metabolic abnormalities

- Pulmonary embolism: tachycardia, T ↓ in V_1–V_4, rarely S in I, Q in III, T inversion in III is seen

- WPW: P-R shortening, wide QRS, and delta wave

Abbreviations: RAE, right atrial enlargement; LAE, left atrial enlargement; LVH, left ventricular enlargement; RVH, right ventricular enlargement.
[a]Normal ECG Intervals and Segment Values.
[b]Use lead II if AVF is isoelectric.
[c](+) → QRS upward deflection > downward deflection.
[d](−) → QRS downward deflection > upward deflection.

TABLE 2–3: BP Management (JNC 7 Guidelines)

A. Hypertension Without Compelling Indications

Goal BP in patient with diabetes or chronic kidney disease < 130/80

Normal BP	Prehypertension
• Systolic < 120 mmHg	• Systolic 120–139 mmHg
• Diastolic < 80 mmHg	• Diastolic 80–89 mmHg
Rx: none needed, TLC	Rx: environmental controls (e.g., smoking), TLC
Stage I HTN	**Stage II HTN**
• Systolic 140–159 mmHg	• Systolic ≥ 160 mmHg
• Diastolic 90–99 mmHg	• Diastolic ≥ 100 mmHg
Rx: thiazide-type diuretics	Rx: 2 drug combination for most patients
• Consider ACE, ARB, β–blocker	• Thiazide diuretics + ACE or ARB
• Calcium channel blocker	• β-Blocker or calcium channel blocker

Abbreviation: TLC, therapeutic lifestyle changes (healthy diet and exercise)
Note: Optimize dosages or add other meds until goal BP is achieved.

TABLE 2–3 (Continued)	
B. Hypertension with Compelling Indications	
• Heart failure	ACE, ARB, thiazide, β-blocker, aldosterone antagonist (K^+ sparing diuretic)
• Post-MI	β-Blocker, ACE, aldosterone antagonist
• High CVD dz. risk	Thiazide, β-blocker, ACE, calcium channel blocker
• Diabetes	ACE, ARB, thiazide, β-blocker, calcium blocker
• Chronic kidney dz.	ACE, ARB
• Recurrent stroke	ACE, thiazide

Source with permission: Chobanian AV, Bakris GL, Black HR, et al. The Seventh Report of the Joint National Committee on Prevention, Detection, Evaluation, and Treatment of High Blood Pressure, the JNC 7 Report, Vol. 289, pp. 2560–2572, 2003.

TABLE 2–4: High Blood Pressure Signs and Symptoms

Life-threatening Conditions	Signs and Symptoms
• Hypertensive encephalopathy	HA, blurry vision
• MI	Chest pain (may not have chest pain in elderly/DM)
• Aortic dissection	Back pain, chest pain
• Neuro	Sensory/motor loss, altered mental status
• Arterial thrombus	Absence of peripheral pulses
• Renal	Decreased urine output
• Eclampsia in pregnancy	Seizure, convulsions

TABLE 2–5: Blood Pressure Classification

	High BP	Urgency	Emergency
BP	>180/110	>180/110	>220/140
Si/Sx	Headache	Severe headache	Chest pain, SOB (shortness of breath)
	Anxiety	SOB	Dysarthria
	Asymptomatic	Edema	Altered consciousness
			Encephalopathy
			Pulmonary edema
			CVA
			Cardiac ischemia

TABLE 2–6: BP Management (Oral Agents)

PO Agents	Dosage	Onset	Duration
Clonidine	0.1–0.2 mg initially then 0.1 mg q1h up to 0.8	30–60 min	6–8 h
Captopril	12.5–25 mg PO tid (may cause hypotension)	15–30 min	4–6 h
Labetalol	200–400 mg PO daily q2-3h	30 min–2 hr	2–12 h
Prazosin	1–2 mg PO q1h	1–2 hr	8–12 h

TABLE 2–7: BP Management (IV Management)

IV Agents	Dosage	Onset	Duration
Nitroprusside	Drip 50 mg in 250 mL D_5W start at 3 µg/kg/min Max: 10 µg/kg/min (check thiocyanate level) Caution: if used >24 h especially in renal failure	Seconds	3–5 min
Esmolol	5 g in 500 mL D_5W, loading dose of 500 µg/kg over 1 min then 50–200 µg/kg/min	1–2 min	10–30 min
Trimethaphan	0.5–5 mg/min (useful in aortic dissection)	1–3 min	10 min
Nicardipine	5 mg/h, increase by 1–2.5 mg/h q15min, max: 15 mg/h	1–5 min	3–6 h
Nitroglycerin	0.25–5 µg/kg/min May develop tolerance	2–5 min	3–5 min
Fenoldopam	0.1–1.6 µg/mg/min May protect renal failure	4–5 min	<10 min
Hydralazine	5–20 mg q20min IV (SE: headache)	10–30 min	2–6 h

TABLE 2–7 (Continued)			
Labetalol	Start at 20 mg → 40 mg → 60 mg → 80 mg; repeat every 10–15 min, max up to 300 mg	5–10 min	3–6 h
Furosemide	10–80 mg (use in conjunction with vasodilator)	15 min	4 h
Enalapril (Vasotec)	1.25–2.5 mg q6h (max 5 mg/24 h), may continue as PO Caution: ↓ dose if CrCl < 30 Cr > 3 or renal stenosis	15 min	>6 h

TABLE 2–8: Cholesterol Classifications (ATP III)

LDL, mg/dL (mmol/L)		Total Cholesterol, mg/dL (mmol/L)	
Optimal	<100 (2.58)	Desirable	<200 (5.17)
Above optimal	100–129 (2.58–3.33)	Borderline high	200–239 (5.17–6.18)
Borderline high	130–159 (3.36–4.11)		
High	160–189 (4.13–4.88)	High	≥240 (6.20)
Very high	≥190(4.91)		
Triglycerides, mg/dL		**HDL, mg/dL**	
Normal	<150	Low	<40
Borderline high	150–199	High	60
High	200–499		
Very high	≥500		

TABLE 2–8 (Continued)			
LDL Goals			
Risk Category	**LDL Goal**	**Initiate TLC**	**Initiate Medication Rx**
0–1 risk factor	<160 mg/dL	≥160 mg/dL	≥190 mg/dL
2+	<130 mg/dL	≥130 mg/dL	≥130 mg/dL (10 years risk 10–20%)
			≥160 mg/dL (10 years risk <10 %)
CHD/CHD risk equivalent	<100 mg/dL	≥100 mg/dL	≥130 mg/dL (100–129 optional)

TLC, therapeutic life style changes (diet and exercise)

CHD Risk Equivalents	**Major Risk Factors Other THAN LDL**
Clinical CHD	Nicotine smoking
Symptomatic carotid artery disease	BP ≥ 140/90 or patient on antihypertensive medication
Diabetes	HDL < 40 mg/dL
Peripheral artery disease	Age (year): ♂ ≥ 45, ♀ ≥ 55
Abdominal aortic aneurysm	Family history of CHD: 1st degree relatives ♂ < 55 years or ♀ < 65 years with MI

(continued)

TABLE 2–8 (Continued)			
Drugs for Management of Hyperlipidemia			
Drug Types	**LDL (%)**	**HDL (%)**	**TG (%)**	**Side Effects and Contra-indications**
HMG-CoA	↓ 18–55	↑ 5–15	↓ 7–30	Myopathy, ↑ LFTs
Nicotinic acids	↓ 5–25	↑ 15–35	↓ 20–50	Hyper-glycemia Hyper-uricemia
				Hepato-toxicity Upper GI distress
				Myositis Pruritus Dry skin
Bile acid sequestrant	↓ 15–30	↑ 3–5	No change	GI distress, ↑ LFTs, and Alk PO$_4$
				Constipation
				↓ Absorption of fat soluble vitamins
Fibric acid	↓ 5–20	↑ 10–20	↓ 20–50	Myopathy Gallstones Dyspepsia

TABLE 2–8 (Continued)				
Fenofibrate	↓ 5–20	↑ 10–20	↓ 20–50	Hepato-toxicity Pancreatitis Rhabdo-myolysis
Ezetimibe (Zetia)	↓ 18	No change	No change	LFTs

Drugs for Management of Hyperlipidemia	
Drug Class	**Indications**
HMG-CoA reductase (statins)	1st line for hyperlipidemia.
	If alone not effective, add Ezetimibe
	If above regimen not effective, D/C them and start atorvastatin/rosuvastatin
	Lovastatin, atorvastatin, and rosuvastatin potentiate effect of warfarin
	Rosuvastatin raises digoxin level
Nicotinic acid (Niacin)	For hyperlipidemia
	For hyperlipidemia + normal to low HDL
Bile acid sequestrant (Cholestyramine)	Mild to moderate ↑ in LDL
	Used in combination with nicotinic acid for severe ↑ LDL
	Impaired absorption: digoxin, warfarin, thiazide, β-blocker, thyroxine, phenobarbital

(continued)

TABLE 2–8 (Continued)	
Fenofibrate	For hypertriglyceridemia and low HDL
	Lowers cyclosporine level
	Potentially nephrotoxic in cyclosporin treated patient
Fibric acid	For hypertriglyceridemia
	Gemfibrozil: potentiates effect of warfarin
	Gemfibrozil absorption property diminished by bile acid sequestering
Ezetimibe (Zetia)	Used for moderate ↑ of LDL
	Most commonly used in combination with statins
	↑ LFTs and alkaline phosphatase when used in combined with statin

Source with permission: NCEP (National Cholesterol Education Program) adult treatment panel III.

TABLE 2–9: Metabolic Syndrome

- At least 3 of the following risk factors

1. Waist circumference: male > 102 cm (>40 in.), female > 88 cm (>35 in.)

2. TG level: ≥150 mg/dL

3. HDL level: male < 40 mg/dL, female < 50 mg/dL

4. Blood pressure: ≥130/85 mmHg

5. Fasting glucose: ≥110 mg/dL

Source with permission: NCEP (National Cholesterol Education Program) adult treatment panel III, U.S. Department of Health and Human Services. NIH publication no. 02-5215, 2002.

TABLE 2–10: Clinical Classification of Chest Pain (ACC)

Typical chest pain

1. Substernal chest discomfort with characteristic quality and duration

2. Chest pain is provoked by exertion or emotional stress

3. Chest discomfort relieved by nitroglycerin

Atypical chest pain

1. Only two of the above characteristics

Noncardiac chest pain

1. Only or none of the above characteristics

Source: ACC (American College of Cardiology).

TABLE 2–11: TIMI Score for UA and NTEMI and Risk of Cardiac Events

Criteria	Score	Risk of Cardiac Events in 14 Days (TIMI 11B)[a]		
		Risk Score	**Death/ MI (%)**	**Death, MI, or Urgent Revascularization(%)**
Age > 65	1	0–1	3	4.7
>3 CAD risk factors (HTN, DM, smoker, ↑cholesterol, FHx of CAD)	1			
Known CAD (stenosis ≥50%)	1	2	3	8.3
Aspirin use in past 7 days	1	3	5	13.2
≥2 angina events in 24 h	1	4	7	19.9
↑ Cardiac markers	1	5	12	26.2
ST ↑ ≥ 0. 5 mm	1	6–7	19	40.9

[a]Entry criteria: UA/NSTEMI defined as ischemic pain at rest within 24 h, with evidence of CAD (ST segment deviation or positive marker).

TABLE 2–12: Acute Myocardial Infarction: Management

1. Nitroglycerine 0.4 mg SL × 3 q5min → if unresponsive give morphine 2 mg IV q5min (hold nitro if SBP < 90)

2. Nitroglycerin ointment 1" to 1 $\frac{1}{2}$" or nitroglycerin patch 0.2–0.6 mg/h q6-8h off qhs (hold nitro if SBP < 90)

3. Aspirin 325 mg crushed then aspirin 162 mg EC PO daily ± Plavix 300 mg × 1 dose then 75 mg PO daily

4. Consider thrombolytic (Alteplase or Reteplase) → if presents within 12 h (check stool guaiac)

5. Consider Integrilin with acute coronary syndrome (non-Q MI and unstable angina) or planned PCI

6. Lopressor 5 mg IV q2-3min × 3 doses → then 25 mg PO q6h (hold if SBP ≤ 90 or HR < 60)
   or Atenolol 5 mg IV, repeated in 5 min followed by 50–100 mg PO daily (hold if SBP ≤ 90 or HR < 60)
   or Esmolol 500 μg/kg over 1 min then 50 μg/kg/min infusion (hold if SBP ≤ 90 or HR < 60)

7. Heparin drip 80–100 unit/kg bolus → follow by → 18 unit/kg or 1000 unit/h (check stool guaiac)
   Check PT/PTT should be 1.5–2 times the control and check 6 h after
   Patient can be started on Lovenox mainly for unstable angina or non-Q-wave MI at 1 mg/kg bid (adjust dose in renal failure : CrCl < 30 mL/min: 1 mg/kg q24h)

8. Nitro-drip (mix 100 mg nitro in 500 mL D_5W). Note → hold if SBP < 90, HR < 60
   Give 15 μg bolus followed by 6 μg/min (2 mL/h)
   Increase by 6 μg/min q5min until → patient is chest pain free, SBP < 100 (max 200 μg/min)

(continued)

TABLE 2–12 (Continued)

9. Acetaminophen (Tylenol) 325–650 mg q4-6h prn for headache

10. Morphine 2–4 mg IV push prn for chest pain if not relieved by nitro

11. Consider ACE (Lisinopril 2.5–5 mg PO daily, titrate to 10–20 mg daily)

12. Lorazepam (Ativan) 1–2 mg PO tid–qid prn for anxiety

13. Consider: atorvastatin 10 mg PO qhs, simvastatin 20 mg PO qhs, pravastatin 40 mg PO qhs
    (consider high-dose statin)

14. Colace 100 mg PO bid for constipation

15. Dimenhydrinate 25–50 mg IV over 2–5 min q4-6h or 50 mg PO q4-5h for nausea

Note

- If heparin induced thrombocytopenia: consider Argatroban 2 μg/kg/min IV continuous infusion.
  Max 10 μg/kg/min, adjust until steady-state aPTT is 1.5–3 times baseline value.

- Avoid using nitro in patient using Viagra and ACE and ASA in pregnant patient.

- Patient with unstable angina → should be started on Lovenox 1 mg/kg bid.

- EF < 40% → patient should be on ACE or ARB or hydralazine and nitrate.

- Be cautious of starting heparin in patient with Hx of cancer due to risk of bleeding.

TABLE 2–12 (Continued)

IIb/IIIa dosing for ACS and planned PCI

- Integrilin bolus of 180 μg/kg (max: 22.6 mg) over 1–2 min then give 2 μg/kg/min (max: 15 mg/h) continue up to 18–24 h or until hospital discharge or

- Aggrestat 10 μg/kg/min → 0.15 μg/kg/min × 18–24 h or

- Reopro 0.25 mg/kg IV then → 0.125 μg/kg/min IV infusion × 12–18 h

The criteria for fibrinolytic therapy

- Onset of symptoms ≤ 3 h can be given up to 12 h (most beneficial if given within 30 min)

- ST segment ↑ of >1 mm in ≥ 2 contiguous ECG limb leads or

- A new left bundle branch block

Absolute contraindications to fibrinolytic therapy

1. Any previous intracranial hemorrhage

2. Documented structural cerebral vascular lesion (e.g., AV malformation)

3. Documented intracranial malignant tumor (primary or metastatic)

4. Ischemic stroke within 3 months with exception of acute ischemic stroke within 3 h

5. Active bleeding or bleeding diathesis (does not include menses)

6. Suspected aortic dissection

7. Significant closed head or facial trauma within 3 months

(continued)

TABLE 2–12 (Continued)

Relative contraindications to fibrinolytic therapy

1. Hx of chronic, severe, poorly controlled hypertension

2. Severe uncontrolled HTN (SBP > 180 or DBP > 110)

3. Hx of prior ischemic stroke > 3 months, dementia, or documented intracranial pathology

4. Active peptic ulcer

5. Pregnancy

6. Traumatic or prolonged CPR (>10 min) or major surgery within < 3 weeks

7. Recent internal bleeding (2–4 weeks)

8. Noncompressible vascular punctures

TABLE 2–13: Heart Failure Signs and Symptoms

Signs	Symptoms
• Weight gain	• Fatigue/exertional dyspnea
• Tachycardia	• SOB
• JVD (jugular venous distention)	• Cough
• Hepatojugular reflux	• Orthopnea
• Lung crackles or wheezes	• PND (paroxysmal nocturnal dyspnea)
• Peripheral edema	• DOE (dyspnea on exertion)
• Hepatomegaly	• Peripheral edema
• S3 (third heart sound)	• Anorexia (severe heart failure)

TABLE 2–14: American College of Cardiology (ACC)/AHA Heart Failure Staging

Stage	
A	Patient with risk factors of heart failure but does not have heart disease
B	Patient with heart disease but does not have symptoms
C	Patient with heart failure symptoms and evidence of heart damage
D	Patient with end-stage disease

Source: ACC/American Heart Association guidelines.

TABLE 2–15: NYHA (New York Heart Association) Classification of Heart Failure

Class	
I	Cardiac disease without resulting limitation of physical activity
II	Comfortable at rest but symptom on activity (fatigue, CP, palpitation)
III	Comfortable at rest but symptom on slight physical activity
IV	Symptoms at rest

TABLE 2–16: ACC/AHA Heart Failure Treatment Recommendations

Stage	Management		
A, B, or C	• Nonpharmacological intervention		
	Limit sodium in diet	Abstain tobacco use	Regular exercise
	Abstain ETOH use	Weight loss (in appropriate setting)	
B	• Start ACE or β-blocker		
C	• Diuretic: if signs of fluid overload		
	• ACE		
	• β-blocker		
	• Digoxin: use in patient not responding to ACE, β-blocker, and diuretic		
	• ARB (angiotensin II receptor antagonist): indicated in patient who cannot tolerate ACE due to cough		
	• Hydralazine + isosorbide: indicated in patient who cannot tolerate ACE due to hypotension, renal insufficiency, or angioedema		
D	• Refer to cardiologist		

Source: American Heart Association guidelines.

TABLE 2–17: Congestive Heart Failure Exacerbation[a]

1. Furosemide 40–80 mg q6-8h

2. β-Blockers/Ca channel blocker (carvedilol, bisoprolol, metoprolol)
   Note: Be cautious of giving β-blockers in patient with COPD. Continue in chronic user.
   Do not use β-blockers in decompensated CHF

3. ACE (e.g., enalapril 2.5 mg PO bid)
   Note: → ACE is contraindicated (creatinine > 3 or CrCl < 30 mL/h).
   → If ACE is contraindicated → consider hydralazine + isosorbide

4. Digoxin 0.5 mg IV/PO × 1 dose followed by 0.25 mg IV × 2 doses then 0.125–0.25 mg daily
   Note: Digoxin is beneficial in patient with A. fib, severe CHF, or EF < 40%.

5. Anticoagulation with heparin or Coumadin (beneficial for patient with EF < 30%)
   Note: Anticoagulation is recommended: severe heart failure and A. fib or Hx of embolism.

6. Inotropic agents (e.g., dobutamine, milrinone, amrinone) are useful if patient is not responding to above regimen or patient awaiting cardiac transplant

TABLE 2–17 (Continued)

Note

- Decompensated CHF → Natrecor: bolus → 2 μg/kg; infusion rate → 0.01 μg/kg/min (contraindicated if SBP < 100).
- Diastolic dysfunction: avoid vigorous diuresis to maintain cardiac output
- Aortic stenosis (AS): avoid ACE in severe AS and use nitrates with precautions
- Hypertrophic obstructive cardiomyopathy (HOCM): avoid vigorous diuresis, digitalis, ACE, hydralazine, and nitrates
- Strict fluid restriction
- Monitor I/O and weight daily
- Avoid using ACE and ASA in pregnant patient

[a]For medication dosage, see Table 2–18.

TABLE 2–18: Commonly Used Drugs in Congestive Heart Failure

Loop Diuretics	Initial Dose	Max. Dose
Bumetanide	0.5–1 mg daily–bid	Titrate to achieve dry weight (up to 10 mg daily)
Furosemide	20–60 mg daily–bid	Titrate to achieve dry weight (up to 400 mg daily)
Torsemide	10–20 mg daily–bid	Titrate to achieve dry weight (up to 200 mg daily)
ACE Inhibitor		
Captopril	6.25 mg tid	50 mg tid
Enalapril	2.5 mg bid	10–20 mg bid
Fosinopril	5–10 mg daily	40 mg daily
Lisinopril	2.5–5 mg daily	20–40 mg daily
Quinapril	10 mg daily	40 mg bid
Ramipril	1.25–2.5 mg daily	10 mg daily

TABLE 2–18 (Continued)		
β-Blocker		
Bisoprolol	1.25 mg daily	10 mg daily
Carvedilol	3.125 mg bid	25 mg bid, if wt > 85 kg → 50 mg bid
Metoprolol tartrate	6.25 mg bid	75 mg bid
Metoprolol succinate	12.5–25 mg daily	200 mg daily
Digitalis Glycosides		
Digoxin	0.125–0.25 mg	0.125–0.25 mg

Note: Monitor potassium when using loop diuretic and keep potassium > 4.

Source: ACC/American Heart Association, Guideline, Evaluation and Management of CHF.

3

Critical Care

TABLE 3–1: Useful Formulas

- A-a gradient (5–15 on room air) = $[(713 \times FiO_2) - (PaCO_2/0.8)] - PaO_2$

- Anion gap (10–15) = $Na^+ - (Cl + HCO_3)$

- Cardiac output (CO) = $HR \times SV$ (4–6 L/min)

- Cardiac index (CI) = $CO \times BSA$ (2.5–3.5 L/min/m^2)

- Ejection fraction (>55%) = (SV/end diastolic volume) $\times$ 100 or

- Ejection fraction = (EDV – ESV)/EDV

- Mean arterial pressure (70–100) = ((2 $\times$ diastolic) + systolic)/3

- Plasma osmolarity (280–290) = $2 \times Na^+$ + (Glu/18) + (BUN/2.8)

- Stroke volume = EDV – ESV

- SVR = 80(MAP – CVP)/CO

TABLE 3–2: ARDS (Acute Respiratory Distress Syndrome)

Definition	Etiology	
Acute onset	Sepsis	Pneumonia
PaO_2/FiO_2 ratio ≤ 200 mmHg	Pancreatitis	Toxins
Chest x-ray $\rightarrow$ bilateral infiltrate	Near-drowning	Inhalation injury
PCWP ≤ 18 mmHg	Multiple trauma with fractures, burns	
	Drugs: IL2, morphine overdose, heroin	
Cardiogenic pulmonary edema vs. ARDS		
• PCWP $\rightarrow$ If $\uparrow$: it is cardiogenic pulmonary edema		
$\rightarrow$ If normal or $\downarrow$: it is ARDS		

TABLE 3–3: Acute Lung Injury

- Bilateral radiographic infiltrates
- A ratio of the partial pressure of arterial oxygen to the fraction of inspired oxygen (PaO_2/FiO_2) between 201 and 300 mmHg, regardless of the level PEEP
- The FiO_2 is expressed as a decimal between 0.21 and 1
- There is no clinical evidence for an elevated left atrial pressure, PCWP is ≤ 18

TABLE 3–4: Burn Injury

Percent Area Assigned to Patient with Burn (Rule of 9s)

Anterior torso	18%	Each arm	9%
Posterior torso	18%	Each leg	18%
Genital area	1%	Head	9%

Fluid Resuscitation in Burn Patient

- Resuscitation fluid = 4 mL/kg × BSA (body surface area burned)

  Include only 2nd and 3rd degree burn in calculation

- Give $1/2$ of total fluid in first 8 h (LR)

- Give $1/2$ of total fluid in next 16 h (LR)

Maintenance Fluid

- 1st 10 kg of total body wt.	- 100 mL/kg/day or 4 mL/kg/h
- 2nd 10 kg of total body wt.	- 50 mL/kg/day or 2 mL/kg/h
- Above 20 kg of total body wt.	- 20 mL/kg/day or 1 mL/kg/h

Example of Fluid Management in Patient with Burn

Resuscitation

- 25 kg child with 20% BSA (2nd degree burn)

- (4 mL × 25 kg) × 20% BSA = 2000 mL/day

- 2000/2 = 1000 → give $1/2$ in 8 h thus 1000/8 → 125 mL/h

(continued)

TABLE 3–4 (Continued)
Maintenance
• 40 mL for the first 10 kg, 20 mL for the second 10 kg, 5 mL for the next 5 kg Total: 65 mL/h
• Hourly infusion for first 8 h Total fluid to be infused: 125 mL/h + 65 mL/h → 190 mL/h
• For next 16 h: 1000 mL/16 h = 62.5 mL/h
• Hourly infusion for next 16 h: 62.5 mL + 65 mL = 127 mL/h

TABLE 3–5: Pulmonary Artery Hypertension	
• Mean pulmonary arterial hypertension (PAP) > 25 mmHg at rest or >30 mmHg during exercise	
• Normal pulmonary capillary wedge pressure	
• Primary (sporadic or familial)	
• Secondary causes	
▪ Congenital systemic pulmonary shunts	▪ HIV
▪ Connective tissue diseases	▪ Persistent pulmonary hypertension of the newborn
▪ Drugs/toxins	▪ Portal hypertension

TABLE 3–6: Hemodynamics in Shock

Type of Shock	CO	PCWP	PAP	CVP	SVR
Cardiogenic	↓	↑	↑	↑	↑
Hypovolemic	↓	↓	↓	↓	↑
Septic	↓	↑	Normal	↓	↓

TABLE 3–7: Noninfectious Causes of Septic Shock

Acute MI	Acute GI hemorrhage
Acute PE	Overzealous diuresis
Acute pancreatitis	Transfusion reaction
Fat emboli syndrome	Adverse drug reaction
Acute adrenal insufficiency	Amniotic fluid emboli

TABLE 3–8: Organ System and Parameters to Follow in Septic Shock

• CNS	Glasgow coma scale
• Respiratory	PaO_2/FiO_2 ratio
• Cardiovascular	Blood pressure via arterial line, pulmonary artery catheter, arterial lactate in hypoperfusion to tissues
• GI	Gastric intramucosal pH, NG aspirate, ileus, lactic acid in bowel ischemia
• Hepatobiliary	Liver function tests, bilirubin, PT/PTT
• Renal	Urine output and serum creatinine
• Hematology/oncology	Platelet count (r/o DIC)

TABLE 3–9: Management of Septic Shock

- Supportive care

- Resuscitation (aggressive IVF, vasopressors)

- Monitoring (see Table 3–8)

- Treat the source of septic shock

- Antibiotic therapy if infectious etiology is suspected (consider broad spectrum Abx)

- Drainage for infection if indicated

- Corticosteroids (stress dose: hydrocortisone 100 mg IV q8h)

- Correction of electrolytes, HCO_3 if pH < 7.1

- Nutrition

TABLE 3–10: Source Control Methods for Common ICU Infection in Addition to Antibiotic Use

Infection Site	Intervention to Control Source of Infection
Catheter-related infection	Removal of catheter
Cholangitis	Bile duct decompression
Endocarditis	Valve replacement
Empyema thoracic	Drainage, decortication
Mediastinitis	Drainage, debridement, and diversion
Pancreatic infection	Drainage or debridement
Peritonitis	Diversion/resection of ongoing source, drainage of abscess, debridement of necrotic tissue
Pneumonia	Chest physiotherapy, suction
Prosthetic valve infection	Device removal
Septic arthritis	Joint drainage and debridement
Sinusitis	Surgical decompression of sinuses
Soft tissue infection	Debridement of necrotic tissue and drainage of abscess
Urinary tract	Relief of obstruction, drainage of abscess, removal or drainage of infected catheter

Source: Marshall, JC, Lowry, SF. Evaluation of the adequacy of source control. In: Sobbald WJ, Vincent JL (eds.), Clinical Trials for the Treatment of Sepsis. Berlin: Springer-Verlag, 1995, p. 329.

TABLE 3–11: Oxygenation Modalities and FiO_2 Relationship

Nasal Cannula O_2	FiO_2	Modality	FiO_2
• 1 L/min	25%	Venturi mask (Venti–Mask)	50%
• 2 L/min	29%	Simple O_2 mask	60%
• 3 L/min	33%	Partial rebreathing mask	75%
• 4 L/min	37%	Nonrebreathing mask	90%
• 5 L/min	41%		

PaO_2 and Saturation Relationship

PaO_2	30	60	75
Saturation	60%	90%	95%

Note

- Venturi mask is useful in patient who are CO_2 retainer; it provides precise administration of O_2.
- $FiO_2 > 60\%$ for more than 3 days can lead to acute tracheobronchitis, and diffuse alveolar damage.
- Oxygenation over 4 L → use humidifier.
- Nasal cannula can support only 6 L of O_2.
- Oxygenation over 6 L → use high flow nasal cannula.

TABLE 3–12: Indication for Placement of Patient on Ventilator

- Respiratory rate > 35

- NIF (negative inspiratory force) ≤ -25

- PaO_2 < 60 mmHg on 60% FiO_2

- $PaCO_2$ > 50 mmHg with pH < 7.20

- Vital capacity < 10–15 mL/kg

- Absent gag or cough reflex

TABLE 3–13: Initial Ventilator Settings

Settings	Normal	Hypoxic	Obstruction Condition	Restrictive Lung Condition
FiO_2	21–100%	100%	40–50%	40–50%
Tidal volume	5–15 L/kg	6 mL/kg	5–7 mL/kg	5–7 mL/kg
Respiratory rate	12–16/min	16–24 min	<24 min	16–24 min
Mode	ACV/SIMV	ACV/SIMV	ACV	ACV/SIMV
PEEP	Minimal	Variable	PEEP dependant	FiO_2/O_2 sat dependant

(continued)

TABLE 3–13 (Continued)

Complications with ventilatory support

- Barotrauma

- Alveolar overdistention

- Hypotension

- Pneumonia

- Atelectasis

- DVT

- GI bleed

- Neuropathy

- Acute sinusitis

Note
• Check CXR after placing patient on ventilator.
• Check ABG in $1/2$ to 1 h after any change in any parameters.
• Hypotension → Rx–IVF.
• Give DVT and GI prophylaxis to all patients on ventilator.
• DVT prophylaxis: Heparin 5000 units Sub Q bid or Lovenox 40 mg Sub Q daily.
• GI prophylaxis: Protonix 40 mg IV daily (bid for GI bleeding)/Pepcid 20 mg IV bid.
• If ABG shows high CO_2 → tidal volume can be increased to blow off CO_2 or ↑ respiratory rate.
• PEEP is useful in hypoxic respiratory failure such as ARDS or cardiogenic pulmonary edema.
• Low levels of PEEP can be used in COPD to keep airways open.
• Increasing PEEP will decrease venous return to the heart and might lead to reductions in BP.
• High levels of TV and PEEP might also predispose patients to barotraumas (vent-induced lung injury).

TABLE 3–14: BIPAP Settings[a]

I = Ventilation	E = Oxygenation
Initial: 10–16	Initial: 6–8
O$_2$ (Oxygenation)	**Respiratory Rate (RR)**
4–10 L or 50–100% (keep < 6 L in COPD)	Initial: 14–20
If CO$_2$ is high: ↑ I or ↑ respiratory rate	If O$_2$ is low: ↑ E or ↑ O$_2$
[a]Use requires patient be alert and cooperative.	

TABLE 3–15: Guidelines for Weaning Patient off the Mechanical Ventilation

1. Patient should be awake and alert (off IV sedation)

2. Consider extubation during daytime due to staffing

3. PEEP $\leq$ 5 cm H_2O

4. ABG $\rightarrow$ $PaCO_2$ acceptable with pH in normal range or their baseline

5. PaO_2 > 60 mmHg on FiO_2 $\leq$ 30%

6. Vital capacity > 10–15 mL/kg (maximum air that can be exhaled after maximum inhalation)

7. Minute ventilation < 10 L/min (total volume of air inhaled and exhaled in 1 min)

8. Respiratory rate < 30/min

9. Peak inspiratory pressure < (–25 cm H_2O)

10. SPTV: >150

11. NIF: < –25, ability to take a deep breath and to generate strong cough reflex to clear secretion

12. Tobin ratio < 100 (respiratory rate/TV (L))

13. Spontaneous ventilation via T-tube for 1–4 h with acceptable blood gases

14. Replace electrolytes (K^+, Mg, PO_4)

TABLE 3–16: Mixed Venous Blood Gas (Normal Values at Sea Level Pressure)

pH 7.32–7.42	$PvCO_2$ 41–51	PvO_2 25–40	HCO_3 28–29	O_2 sat 60–85%
Note				

- The pH difference between arterial blood and venous blood is 0.03–0.04.

- $PvCO_2 < PaCO_2 \rightarrow$ means there is contamination by pulmonary capillary blood.

- If venous oxygen sat is < 65% → means increased unloading of oxygen in periphery, usually due to incomplete resuscitation, shock, or advanced disease process.

TABLE 3–17: ABG (Normal Values)

pH 7.35–7.45	$PaCO_2$ 35–45	PaO_2 80–100	HCO_3 22–28	O_2 saturation >97%
Note				

- ΔCO_2 10 → ΔpH 0.08; ΔpH 0.10 → ΔK^+ 0.5 meq/L (inversely proportional).

- The arterial and venous pH difference is 0.01–0.03. It is in patient with CHF and shock.

- pH of 7.15 is an indication for HCO_3 infusion.

TABLE 3–18: ABG and Respiratory and Metabolic Disturbance	
Metabolic acidosis	1 mmol/L HCO_3 ↓ = ΔPCO_2 1–1.3
	PCO_2 = last 2 digits of pH
Metabolic alkalosis	1 mmol/L HCO_3 = ΔPCO_2 0.6–0.7
	PCO_2 = 0.9(HCO_3) + 9
Respiratory acidosis (acute)	↑ PCO_2 of 10 = 1 mmol/L ↓ of HCO_3
Respiratory acidosis (chronic)	↑ PCO_2 of 10 = 3–3.5 mmol/L ↓ of HCO_3
Respiratory alkalosis (acute)	↓ PCO_2 of 10 = 2–2.5 mmol/L ↓ HCO_3
Respiratory alkalosis (chronic)	↓ PCO_2 of 10 = 4–5 mmol/L ↓ HCO_3

TABLE 3–19: ABG and Appropriate Compensation	
Metabolic acidosis	PCO_2 = 1.5(HCO_3) + 8(±2)
Metabolic alkalosis	Δ ↑ 1 HCO_3 = Δ ↑ 0.7 PCO_2
Respiratory acidosis (acute)	Δ10 PCO_2 = Δ1 HCO_3
Respiratory acidosis (chronic)	Δ10 ↑ PCO_2 = Δ ↑ 3–3.5 HCO_3
Respiratory alkalosis (acute)	Δ2 meq/L HCO_3 ↓ = 10 mmHg ΔCO_2
Respiratory alkalosis (chronic)	Δ4 meq/L HCO_3 ↓ = 10 mmHg ΔPCO_2

TABLE 3–20: Metabolic Alkalosis	
Etiologies	**Workup**
• Volume depletion (diuretic use, GI loss, dehydration)	• BUN/Cr • U_{Cl} (urine chloride level)
• Compensation from hypercapnia	• Aldosterone level
• 1st degree hyperaldosteronism (Conn's syndrome)	
• 2nd degree hyperaldosteronism	
• Cushing's syndrome	
Chloride Responsive (Urine Chloride < 15 meq/L)	**Chloride Resistant (Urine Chloride > 25 meq/L)**
• GI loss	• Potassium depletion
• Diuretics	• Mineralocorticoid excess
• Volume depletion	
• Posthypercapnia	

TABLE 3–20 (Continued)	
Anion Gap (AG) (10–15) = $Na^+ - (Cl + HCO_3)$	
$\Delta AG/\Delta HCO_3$	$\Delta AG \approx \Delta HCO_3 \rightarrow$ purely anion gap metabolic acidosis
ΔAG = calculated AG – 12	$\Delta AG < \Delta HCO_3 \rightarrow$ AG + non-AG metabolic acidosis
ΔHCO_3 = 24 – Pt HCO_3	$\Delta AG > \Delta HCO_3 \rightarrow$ metabolic acidosis + metabolic alkalosis
• ↓ Albumin 1 g = ↓ anion gap 2.2–2.5	

TABLE 3–21: Metabolic Acidosis and Anion Gap

Normal Anion Gap Metabolic Acidosis	↑ Anion Gap Metabolic Acidosis
HARDUP C	**MUDPILES**
• Hyperalimentation (TPN)	• Methanol
• Adrenal insufficiency	• Uremia, renal failure
• Acetazolamide (carbonic anhydrase inhibitor)	• Diabetic ketoacidosis (DKA)
• Renal tubular acidosis (RTA)	• Paraldehyde
• Diarrhea	• INH, iron
• Ureteroenterostomy	• Lactic acid/alcoholic ketoacidosis
• Pancreatic fistula	• Ethylene glycol
• Small bowel fistula	• Salicylic acid intoxication (ASA)
• Extra chloride	

TABLE 3–21 (Continued)	
Workup	
• Urine anion gap (UAG)	• Urine ketones
• Urine NH_4	• Serum β-hydroxybutyrate
• If urine AG (−) and urine NH_4	• BUN/creatinine
→ type II RTA, GI cause, extra acid	• Lactic acid
• If urine AG (+) and urine ↑ NH_4	• Osmolal gap
→ Type I/IV RTA	• Toxins (check urine and serum)
• ? Serum renin level (type V RTA)	• Serum aldosterone level (type V RTA)
↓ Anion Gap	
• Paraproteinemia (multiple myeloma)	• Hyperchloremia (bromide toxicity)
• Hyponatremia	• Hypermagnesemia
• Hypercalcemia	• Hyperkalemia
• Lithium	• Polymyxin B
• Hypoalbuminemia (anion gap decreases 2.5 per 1 g/dL decrease in albumin)	

TABLE 3–22: Urine Anion Gap (UAG): Useful in Evaluation of Patient with Hyperchloremic Metabolic Acidosis

Urine anion gap = urine Na^+ + urine K^+ – urine chloride

Differential Diagnosis of Hyperchloremic Metabolic Acidosis			
Condition	Urine Anion Gap	Plasma K^+	Urine pH
Normal, exogenous ammonium chloride	(−)	Normal	<5.5
Gastrointestinal HCO_3 loss	(−)	↓/Normal	>5.5
Distal RTA	(+)	↓/Normal	>5.5
Hyperkalemic distal RTA	(+)	↑	>5.5
Primary aldosterone deficiency	(+)	↑	<5.5
Note			
• If gap is (+) → renal HCO_3 loss → distal RTA or 1st degree aldosterone deficiency.			
• If gap is (−) → normal or GI HCO_3 loss.			

TABLE 3–23: Osmolal Gap

Plasma osmolarity (280–290) = $2 \times Na^+ + (Glu/18) + (BUN/2.8)$

Osmolal gap (<10) = measured plasma osmolarity by lab − calculated plasma osmolarity

Osmolal Gap ↑ in Following

• Ethanol	• Hyperproteinemia/hyperlipidemia
• Ethylene glycol	• Chronic renal failure
• Isopropyl alcohol	• Sorbitol
• Methanol	• X-ray dye

TABLE 3–24: A-a gradient

- 5–15 mmHg on room air; 60–70 mmHg on 100% O_2; 15–25 mmHg in elderly

Note
- A-a gradient ↑ 6 mmHg for every 10% ↑ in FiO_2.
- When hypoxia is due to hypoventilation, A-a gradient remains normal.

↓ PaO_2 and ↑ A-a Gradient

Diffusion Impairment	Shunt (Does Not Improve with O_2)
- Collagen vascular lung dz. (IPF)[a]	- Atelectasis
- Interstitial lung dz. (Sarcoid)	- Cardiac R → L shunt (septal defect)
V–Q Mismatch (Improves with O_2)	- Pulmonary hemorrhage
- Asthma	- Pneumonia
- COPD	- Pulmonary A-V fistula
- Pulmonary emboli	- Pulmonary edema
Diffusion Barrier	- ARDS
- ARDS	- Congestive heart failure

[a]IPF, interstitial pulmonary fibrosis.

TABLE 3–25: Pulmonary Artery Reading (Swan Reading)

RA pressure = 0–8 mmHg	Central venous pressure = 2–8 mmHg
RV pressure systolic/diastolic = 15–30/2 mmHg	CO = 4–6 L/min
PA pressure systolic/diastolic = 15–30/5–12 mmHg	PCWP = 2–10 mmHg
Mean pulmonary artery pressure = 5–10 mmHg	SVR = 800–1200 dynes/s/cm^5
Cardiac index = 2.5–3.5 L/min/m^2	Ejection fraction = >55%
PCWP = pulmonary capillary wedge pressure	SVR = systemic vascular resistance
PCWP = left ventricle end diastolic volume (LVEDV)	CO = cardiac output
PAP = pulmonary artery pressure	CVP = central venous pressure

4
Endocrinology

TABLE 4–1: Electrolyte Corrections and Formulas

- Corrected Na^+ for glucose = $Na^+ + [(Glu - 100) \times 0.016]$
- Corrected Na^+ for glucose = $Na^+ + [(Glu - 200)/42]$
- For each 100 ↑ glucose → Na^+ ↓ by ≈1.6
- Corrected HCO_3 for anion gap = HCO_3 + (anion gap – 12)
- Anion gap (10–15) = $Na^+ - (Cl + HCO_3)$
- ↓ Albumin of 1 g = ↓ anion gap by ≈ 2.2 – 2.5
- Plasma osmolarity (280–290) = $2 \times Na^+ + (Glu/18) + (BUN/2.8)$

TABLE 4–2: Blood Sugar

	Normal (mg/dL)	Prediabetes (mg/dL)	Diabetes (mg/dL)
Fasting plasma sugar[a]	<100	100–125	≥126
Oral glucose tolerance test	<140	140–199	≥200

[a]Fasting plasma sugar needs to be repeated once to diagnose patient with DM.
Source with permission: Reprinted with permission from American Diabetes Association, 2005. Available at: http://www.diabetes.org.

TABLE 4–3: Insulin Types			
Bolus or mealtime insulin	**Onset**	**Peak**	**Duration**
Lispro (Humalog)	10–15 min	30–90 min	4–6 h
Aspart (NovoLog)	10–20 min	1–3 h	3–5 h
Regular (Humulin R, Novolin R)	30–60 min	2–4 h	8–12 h
Regular buffered (Velosulin)	30–60 min	1–3 h	8 h
Basal insulin			
NPH (Humulin N, Novolin N)	1–2 h	4–12 h	16–24 h
Lente (Humulin L, Novolin L)	1–3 h	7–15 h	16–24 h
Ultralente (Humulin U Ultralente)	4–8 h	10–30 h	≈ 36 h
Glargine (Lantus)	4–8 h	No peak	20–24 h
Combination			
75/25 (NPL/Lispro, Humalog 75/25)	15 min	30–90 h	24 h
70/30 (NPH/Aspart, NovoLog 70/30)	15–30 min	1–4 h	24 h
50/50 (NPH/regular)	30–60 min	4–8 h	24 h

(continued)

TABLE 4–3 (Continued)			
70/30 (NPH/regular, Humulin R 70/30/Novolin R 70/30)	30–60 min	4–8 h	24 h

Abbreviations: NPH, Neutral Protamine Hagedorn; NPL, Neutral Protamine Listro.

Note: Patient with renal insufficiency: studies have shown increased circulating levels of insulin thus careful glucose monitoring and dose adjustments of insulin may be necessary.

TABLE 4–4: Glucose and Insulin

- Usual insulin daily requirement: 0.5 unit/kg/day

- Insulin daily requirement in renal insufficiency: 0.2–0.4 unit/kg/day

- Glargine insulin standing dose is 0.1–0.2 unit/kg/day

- Usual insulin dosing: 2/3 in AM (1/3 regular and 2/3 NPH); 1/3 in PM (1/3 regular and 2/3 NPH)

- Rx for level >200 → Rx → insulin sliding scale: 150–200 → 2 units regular
  - 201–250 → 4 units
  - 251–300 → 6 units
  - 301–350 → 8 units
  - 351–400 → 10 units
  - >400 → 12 units and call MD

Note: Above insulin sliding scale varies from institute to institute.

TABLE 4–5: Diabetic Ketoacidosis (DKA)

1. Normal saline (NS) 1st liter should be given quickly then 1 L/h until fluid deficit is corrected then start maintenance fluid 150–500 mL/h (usual fluid deficit: 6–8 L)
   Note: If hypernatremia is noted start with 0.45% saline initially.

2. Monitor glucose q1h initially for first 2–3 h and then q2-4h for next 12 h

3. Monitor (K, anion gap, HCO_3) q2h (correct sodium for glucose)

4. Change IVF to D_5NS or D_5 ½ NS once the glucose level reaches 250–300 mg/dL

5. Insulin regular 10–15 units IV (0.2 unit/kg) followed by infusion of 5–10 unit/h, 0.1 unit/kg/h
   (Infusion → 100 units in 500 mL NS → infusion rate 50 mL/h gives 10 unit/h)
   Note: An appropriate response to insulin Rx is: ↓ blood glucose of 50–75 mg/dL/h.

6. ↓ Insulin infusion rate to 2–3 unit/h → when glucose level ↓ to 250–300 mg/dL

Note: Stop insulin infusion when anion gap normalizes (10–15) and HCO_3 is close to normal, give Sub Q insulin prior to stopping infusion (IV insulin ½ life is only few minutes)

K^+: Potassium replacement → K^+ should ↓ with insulin Rx thus → add 20–40 meq KCl to each liter of IVF and then Δ to K-phosphate to prevent chloride overload (monitor potassium q2h); vigorously replace K^+ → give KCl via IV (10 meq/h) or central line (20 meq/h) or NG tube

(continued)

TABLE 4–5 (Continued)

7. PO_4: If PO_4 is < 1.5 meq/L → phosphorus 2.5–5 mg/kg in 500 mL over 6 h

Mg: Replacement is only required if severe hypomagnesemia, refractory hypokalemia or patient with ventricular arrhythmia → Rx: magnesium sulfate 2.5–5 mg IV

HCO_3: Routine use is not required unless patient pH ≤ 7.15 → Rx: add 50–100 meq HCO_3 to each liter (50–100 mmol $NaHCO_3$ in 200–400 mL NS/D_5W at 200 mL/h)

TABLE 4–6: Nonketotic Hyperosmolar Syndrome (NKHS)

1. Fluid replacement and electrolyte replacement is essential in management

2. Calculate fluid deficit and replace

3. Monitor glucose q1h initially for first 2–3 h and then q2-4h for next 12 h

4. Monitor electrolytes q2h (correct sodium for glucose and calculate serum osmolarity)

5. NS → 1–1.5 L/h initially then change to $\frac{1}{2}$ NS at 500 mL/h (↓ rate in patient with CHF)

6. Regular insulin 5–10 units should be given initially in severe hyperglycemia (>600)

7. Infusion → 5–10 unit/h (50 units of regular insulin in 500 mL of NS at 50 mL/h → gives 5 unit/h)

When glucose reaches 250–300 mg/dL → ↓ infusion rate to 1–2 unit/h and change IVF to D_5 $\frac{1}{2}$ NS

8. After stopping infusion → place patient on sliding scale and regular insulin Sub Q

K^+: Potassium replacement → should be expected with insulin Rx → add 20–40 meq KCl to each liter of IVF and then Δ to K-phosphate to prevent chloride overload (monitor potassium q2h); vigorously replace K^+ → give KCl via IV (10 meq/h) or central line (20 meq/hr) or NG

9. PO_4: If PO_4 is < 1.5 meq/L → phosphorus 2.5–5 mg/kg in 500 mL over 6 h

Note: Monitor urinary output.

TABLE 4–7: Thyroid Function Tests (Normal Values)				
TSH	**Total T_3**	**Total T_4**	**Free T_4**	**Radioactive Iodide Uptake (I^{123})**
0.3–5 μU/mL	95–190 ng/dL	5–12 μg/dL	Variable	10–30%

TABLE 4–8: Thyroid Diseases and Lab Findings					
	TSH	**Total T_3**	**Total T_4**	**Free T_4**	**RAIU**
Hyperthyroidism	↓	↑	↑	↑	↑
1st degree hypothyroidism	↑	N	↓	↓	N or ↓
2nd degree hypothyroidism	↓	N	↓	↓	N or ↓
Subclinical hypothyroidism	↑	N	N	N	N
Subclinical hyperthyroidism	↓	N	N	N	N
Sick euthyroid syndrome	N/↓	↓	N	N	

Abbreviations: RAIU: radioactive iodide uptake (I^{123}).

TABLE 4–9: Thyroiditis and RAIU Relationship	
High RAIU	**Low RAIU**
Hashitoxicosis	Subacute granulomatosis (de Quervain's thyroiditis)
	Radiation–palpation–drug-induced thyroiditis
	Subacute lymphocytic thyroiditis
	Chronic lymphocytic thyroiditis
	Postpartum thyroiditis
	Hashimoto's thyroiditis

TABLE 4–10: Diagnostic Criteria for Thyroid Storm

Signs and Symptoms	Score	Signs and Symptoms	Score
Tachycardia → 99–109	5	CNS → Mild agitation	10
110–119	10	Moderate → delirium	20
120–129	15	→ Psychosis	
130–139	20	Extreme lethargy	
>140	25	Severe seizure/coma	30
Temp → 99–99.9	5	CHF → Mild pedal edema	5
100–100.9	10	Moderate bibasilar rales	10
101–101.9	15	Severe pulmonary edema	15
102–102.9	20	A-Fib	10
103–103.9	25	Precipitant history	
>104	30	→ Negative	0

TABLE 4–10 (Continued)			
GI → moderate. N/V/D, abdominal pain	10	→ Positive	10
Severe unexplained jaundice	20		

Note: <25: storm is unlikely; 25–44: supports the Dx of storm; ≥45: highly suggestive of storm.

Source with permission: Burch HB, Wartofsky L. Life-threatening thyrotoxicosis: thyroid storm. *Endocrinol Metab Clin North Am* 1993; 22:263–277.

TABLE 4–11: Etiology of SIADH	
Medications	**CNS Causes**
Amiodarone	Brain abscess
Carbamazepine	Encephalitis
Chlorpromazine	Head trauma
Chlorpropamide	Hydrocephalus
Cyclophosphamide	Meningitis
Cytoxan	Pituitary surgery
Oxcarbazepine	Psychosis
Oxytocin	Stroke
Phenothiazine	Subdural hematoma
SSRI	Tumor (brain)
Theophylline	
Tricyclic antidepressants	
Vincristine	

TABLE 4–11 (Continued)	
Pulmonary Etiology	**Carcinomas**
Asthma	Bronchogenic cancer
Bronchiectasis	Lymphoma
COPD	Mesothelioma
Empyema/abscess	Neuroblastoma
Pneumonia	Pancreatic cancer
Pneumothorax	Prostate cancer
Positive pressure ventilation	Small cell lung carcinoma
Tuberculosis	Thymoma
Management of SIADH	
• Correct underlying cause	
• Fluid restriction: 500–800 L/day	
• Loop diuretic: furosemide 40 mg IV q6h with NaCl IVF replacement	
• Slowly correct sodium (see Table 8–2)	
• Demeclocycline 600–1200 mg PO daily	

TABLE 4–12: Etiology of Diabetes Insipidus	
Central	**Nephrogenic**
Cerebral hemorrhage	Cidofovir
CNS malignancy/infection	Demeclocycline
Idiopathic	Foscarnet
Head trauma	Hypercalcemia
Hypoxic encephalopathy	Hypokalemia
Sheehan's syndrome	Lithium toxicity
	Osmotic diuresis
	Papillary necrosis
Management of DI	
• Central DI	
• Intranasal DDAVP	
• Nephrogenic DI	
• Thiazide diuretic	

TABLE 4–13: Adrenal Crisis	
Signs and symptoms	
Nausea/vomiting/dehydration	Anorexia → weight loss
Abdominal pain → acute abdomen	Unexplained fever
Hyperpigmentation or vitiligo	Weakness/malaise
Constipation/diarrhea	Syncope
Labs/studies	
• CBC	• BMP
• Random and 24 h urinary cortisol level	• Calcium
• TSH, T_3, T_4	• CXR
• HIV testing	• CT Abd
• Adrenocorticotropic hormone stimulation test (see below)	• CT Head
	• ECG
Lab evaluation	
Hypotension	Unexplained hypoglycemia
Hyponatremia	Hyperkalemia
Hypercalcemia	Azotemia
Eosinophilia	↑ TSH, and ↓ T_3, T_4
ECG →	CT Abd → calcification/hemorrhage of adrenal gland
Peaked T waves	CT Head → destruction of pituitary/mass lesion

(continued)

TABLE 4–13 (Continued)

Management

1. Treat hypotension with NS or D_5NS (2–3 L) 500 mL/h to wide open

2. Correct electrolytes

3. Dexamethasone sodium phosphate 4 mg IV or hydrocortisone 100 mg IV q6-8h for 1st 24 h
   Note: Dexamethasone is preferred over hydrocortisone because it does not interfere with ACTH stimulation test.

4. Fludrocortisone 0.1–0.2 mg/day

5. Steroid dose should be adjusted during stress (infection, surgery, and so on)

Adrenocorticotropic hormone stimulation test

1. Obtain baseline serum cortisol and ACTH levels

2. Administer 0.25 mg of cosyntropin (synthetic ACTH) IV/IM

3. Repeat cortisol levels every 30–60 min and 6 h after ACTH administration

4. Normal response is indicated when the cortisol level doubles in response to ACTH stimulation

5. In adrenal insufficiency, serum cortisol levels fail to rise after ACTH administration

TABLE 4–14: Hyperparathyroidism	
Signs and Symptoms	
Anemia	Nephrolithiasis
Hypophosphatemia	Bone disease
Hypomagnesemia	Proximal/distal RTA
Hyperuricemia	↑ Production of calcitriol
Weakness and fatigue	Muscle weakness
Constipation	↑ Gastrin production → peptic ulcer
Pancreatitis	Nephrogenic diabetes insipidus
Shortening of Q-T interval	Corneal calculi deposition
PTH inhibit proximal tubular bicarbonate reabsorption → mild metabolic acidosis	
CNS dysfunction	

(continued)

TABLE 4–14 (Continued)

Management

- Treat hypercalcemia (also see Chapter 8)

- IVF → NS at 200–300 mL/h and adjust to maintain the urine output to 100–150 mL/h

- Furosemide diuretic

- Calcitonin

- Corticosteroids

- Pamidronate (if serum calcium is > 13.5 mg/dL (3–3.4 mg/dL) consider 60 mg IV)

- Zoledronic acid 4 mg IV over 15 min

- Etidronate/clodronate/risedronate

- Gallium nitrate 200 mg IV continuous infusion for 5 days (SE: nephrotoxicity)

- Chelation therapy with EDTA

- Dialysis

5
Gastroenterology

TABLE 5–1: Etiologies of Pancreatitis

Gall stones	Alcohol	Hyperlipidemia (I, IV, V)
Hypercalcemia	Trauma	Atheroembolism
Pancreatic cancer	Duodenal stricture/ obstruction	Ampullary stenosis
Post-ERCP	α-1-Antitrypsin deficiency	Pregnancy
Vasculitis	Scorpion venom	Choledochocele
Medications Associated with Pancreatitis		
Thiazides	Furosemide	Didanosine
Estrogen	Azathioprine	L-Asparaginase
Metronidazole	Pentamidine	Salicylate (Aspirin)
Tetracycline	Sulindac	Valproic acid
Sulfasalazine	Protease inhibitor	
Infections Associated with Pancreatitis		
Ascaris	Aspergillus	CMV/EBV
Coxsackie	Cryptosporidium	Hepatitis A & B
HIV	HSV	Legionella
Leptospira	Mycoplasma	Mumps/rubella
Salmonella	Toxoplasmosis	Varicella–zoster

TABLE 5–1 (Continued)		
Diagnostic Labs and Studies for Pancreatitis		
Amylase	Lipase[a]	Abd ultrasound
BMP with Mg level	Calcium level	?Hep B surface Ag
Lipid panel	?PT/PTT/INR	?UA
LFT, bilirubin, alk PO_4	?Blood C&S	?Urine/serum Tox screen
α-1-Antitrypsin deficiency		
[a]Lipase: 94% sensitive, 96% specific.		

TABLE 5–2: Ranson's Criteria	
0 Hour	**48 Hours**
• Give one point for each positive finding	
• Age > 55 years	• HCT—fall by ≥10%
• WBC > 16,000/mm^3	• BUN ↑ by ≥ 5 mg/dL (1.8 mmol/L)
• Glucose > 200 mg/dL (11.1 mmol/L)	• Calcium < 8 meq/L (2 mmol/L)
• LDH > 350 IU/L	• PaO$_2$ < 60 mmHg
• AST > 250 IU/L	• Base deficit > 4 meq/L
• ALT > 80 IU/L	• Fluid sequestration > 6 L
Prognosis	
Total Score	**Mortality**
≤2	<5%
3–4	15–20%
5–6	40%
≥7	>99%

TABLE 5–2 (Continued)

Acute Pancreatitis: Management

- Vigorous fluid replacement (NS 3–5 L over 2–3 h then →
  D_5NS or NSS at 125–150 mL/h)

- Pain management
  - → Fentanyl 50–100 µg/dose every 1–2 h as needed or
  - → Morphine 2–5 mg IV q3-4h or
  - → Meperidine 50–100 mg IV/IM q4h prn (caution in
    elderly due to risk of delirium)
    GFR 10–50 mL/min, 75% of normal dose at normal
    intervals
    GFR less than 10 mL/min, 50% of normal dose at usual
    intervals

- Ranitidine 50 mg IV q6-8h or Famotidine 20 mg IV q12h

- If there is necrotizing pancreatitis (involving more than
  30% of the pancreas), initiate antimicrobial therapy with
  Primaxin 0.5–1 g IV q6h continue for >7 days

- If infected pseudocyst or abscess: → Timentin 3.1 g IV or
  → Unasyn 3 g IV q6h or
  → Primaxin 0.5–1 g IV
  q6h

- Consider CT guided aspiration if no improvement with
  Abx therapy

TABLE 5–3: Viral Hepatitis	
Hepatitis A	
Transmission	Fecal–oral route
Incubation period	2–6 weeks
Diagnosis	Acute hepatitis: (+) IgM anti-HAV
	Prior exposure: (+) IgG anti-HAV
Rx	Supportive
Prevention	Hep A vaccine
Hepatitis B	
Transmission	Sexual and parenteral
Incubation period	2–6 months
Diagnosis	See below

Hepatitis B Lab Interpretations

	HBs Ag	Anti-HBs	Anti-HBc	IgM Anti-HBc
Susceptible	−	−	−	
Immune due to vaccination	−	+	−	
Immune due to natural infection	−	+	+	
Acute infection (≤6 months)	+	−	+	+

TABLE 5–3 (Continued)				
Chronic infection	+	–	+	–
Rx: Acute	Supportive			
Chronic	Interferon-α-2b or lamivudine or adefovir dipivoxil			
Prevention	Hep B vaccine (series of 3 shots)			
Hepatitis C				
Transmission	Percutaneous and sexual			
Incubation period	1–3 months			
Diagnosis	Acute hepatitis: (+) HCV RNA ± anti-HCV			
	Chronic hepatitis: (+) HCV RNA (+) anti-HCV			
	Resolved hepatitis: (–) HCV RNA ± anti-HCV			
Rx	Interferon-α-2b			
	Interferon-α-2b + ribavirin			
	PEG–interferon-α-2a + ribavirin			
	Liver transplant			
Prevention	No vaccination available			

(continued)

TABLE 5–3 (Continued)	
Hepatitis D	
Transmission	Percutaneous and sexual (occurs in patient with HBsAg (+) patients)
Incubation period	?
Diagnosis	Anti-HDV total, anti-HDV IgM, serum HD Ag, serum HDV
	RNA, HbsAg ?
Rx	Interferon-α and transplant
Prevention	Immunization with Hep B → Hep B vaccine (series of 3 shots)
Hepatitis E	
Transmission	Fecal–oral route
Incubation period	?
Diagnosis	HEV-Ag RNA, IgM, and IgG assays
Rx	Supportive care
Prevention	HEV vaccine

TABLE 5–4: Inflammatory Bowel Disease (Crohn's Vs. UC)

	Crohn's Disease (CD)	Ulcerative Colitis (UC)
Anatomical site		
Esophagus	Uncommon	Not seen
Stomach/duodenum	Uncommon	Not seen
Jejunum	Uncommon	Not seen
Ileum	2/3 of patients	Not seen
Colon	2/3 of patients	Common
Perineal dz.	Common	Not seen
Clinical features		
Abdominal pain	Common	Variable
Abdominal mass	Common	Absent
Diarrhea	Very common	Rare
Fever	Common	Common
Growth failure in kids	Common	Rare
Malnutrition	Common	Rare
Rectal bleed	Rare	Very common
Weight loss	Common	Rare

(continued)

TABLE 5–4 (Continued)		
Complications		
Cancer	Common	Very common
Fistula	Common	Absent
Perforation	Not seen	Unknown
Stricture	Common	Unknown
Toxic megacolon	Absent	Unknown
Lab finding		
Perinuclear-staining antineutrophil cytoplasmic antibodies	Present	Present
Anti-*Saccharomyces cerevisiae* antibodies	Present	
Endoscopic finding		
Aphthous ulcers	Common	Absent
Cobble stoning	Common	Absent
Friability	Common	Very common
Pseudo polyps	Common	Common
Rectal involvement	Very common	Common
Radiologic finding		
Distribution	Segmented	Continuous
Fissures	Common	Absent

TABLE 5–4 (Continued)		
Fistula	Common	Rare
Ileal involvement	Nodular, narrowed	Dilated
Stricture	Common	Rare
Ulceration	Deep with submucosal involvement	Superficial (fine)
Management of CD and UC			

Disease Severity	CD	Distal UC	Extensive UC
Mild	Amino-salicylate PO	Amino-salicylate PO/PR	Amino-salicylate PO
	Metronidazole PO Budesonide or Ciprofloxacin PO	Cortico-steroids PR	
Moderate	Corticosteroids PO	Amino-salicylate PO, PR	Amino-salicylate PO
	Azathioprine or Mercaptopurine PO	Cortico-steroids PR	

(continued)

TABLE 5–4 (Continued)			
Severe	Cortico-steroids PO/parenteral	Cortico-steroids PO/PR/ parenteral	Cortico-steroids PO/ parenteral
	Methotrexate IV, Sub Q		Cyclosporine IV
	Infliximab IV		
Refractory	Infliximab IV	Cortico-steroids PO, IV	Cortico-steroids PO/IV
		Azathioprine or Mercapto-purine PO	Azathioprine or Mercapto-purine PO
Perianal disease	Metronidazole or		
	Ciprofloxacin PO		
	Infliximab IV		
	Azathioprine or		
	Mercaptopurine PO		

- Sulfasalazine should always be supplemented with folate, little absorbed in small intestine
- Pentasa: time released, absorbed in small intestine
- Asacol: due to pH of 7, it is well absorbed in terminal small bowel and ileum

TABLE 5–5: *H. pylori* Treatment

Regimen A	PPI + amoxicillin 1000 mg + Clarithromycin 500 mg (take each medication twice daily for 2 wks)
Regimen B	PPI + Metronidazole 500 mg + Clarithromycin 500 mg (take each medication twice daily for 2 wks)
Regimen C	RBC 400 mg + Clarithromycin 500 mg + (Amoxicillin 1000 mg OR Metronidazole 500 mg OR Tetracycline 500 mg) (take each medication twice daily for 2 wks)
Regimen D	PPI qd + Bismuth subsalicylate 525 mg qid + Metronidazole 500 mg tid + Tetracycline 500 mg qid (take each medication for 2 wks)
Regimen E	Bismuth subsalicylate 525 mg qid + Metronidazole 250 mg qid + Tetracycline 500 mg qid + H2 receptor antagonist (take each medication twice daily for 2 wks except H2 give for 4 wks)

PPI = Lansoprazole 30 mg OR Omeprazole 20 mg

RBC = Ranitidine bismuth citrate

Source with permission: Colin Howden, Richard Hunt, American journal of gastroenterology, Guidelines for management of *H. pylori* infection, 1998,93;12.

TABLE 5–6: Paracentesis	
Tube Number	**Test**
1	Bacterial and fungal C&S
2	Albumin, LDH, and protein
3	Cell count and differential
4	Cytology

TABLE 5-7: Ascitic Fluid Analysis

Essential Tests	Optional Tests	Unusual Tests
• Cell count with Diff	• Glucose	• TB smear
• Albumin	• LDH	• Cytology
• Culture	• Amylase	
• Total protein	• Gram stain	
• Serum albumin		

If cell count > 250/mm^3 → most likely → bacterial peritonitis (Rx: see Chapter 7)

SAAG (Serum-Ascites Albumin Gradient) = Serum Albumin – Ascites Albumin

>1.1 (Secondary to Portal HTN)	<1.1 (Secondary to Other than Portal HTN)
• ETOH hepatitis	• Nephrotic syndrome
• ↑ Right heart pressure	• Ischemic bowel
• Cirrhosis	• Pancreatic ascites

(continued)

113

TABLE 5-7 (Continued)

- Massive mets to liver
- Budd-Chiari syndrome
- Myxedema (iodine)
- Occlusion of portal vein

- Peritoneal carcinoma
- Tuberculosis of peritoneum

Transudates

Condition	CHF	Cirrhosis	Nephrotic Syndrome
SAAG	>1.1	>1.1	<1.1
Protein	<2.5 g/dL	<3 g/dL	<2.5 g/dL
Glucose	WNL	WNL	WNL
WBC	WNL (<250 μL)	WNL	WNL
RBC	Few	Few	Few

Exudates

Condition	Bacterial Peritonitis	Tuberculous Peritonitis	Pancreatitis	Malignancy	Chylous
SAAG	<1.1	<1.1	<1.1	<1.1	
Protein	>3 g/dL	>3 g/dL	>2.5 g/dL	>3 g/dL	>2.5 g/dL
Glucose	<60 mg/dL	<60 mg/dL	WNL	<60 mg/dL	WNL
WBC	>500, PMN	>500, MN	>500	>500	Few
RBC	Few	Few	Few	Many	Few

6
Hematology/Oncology

TABLE 6–1: Blood Products	
• Hct = Hb × 3	• 1 Unit of FFP = 200 mL
• 1 Unit of PRBC → ↑ Hb by 1 g/dL	• 1 Unit of cryoprecipitate → ↑ fibrinogen 5–10 mg/dL
• 1 Unit of PRBC → ↑ Hct by 3%	
• 1 Unit of platelet → ↑ by 10,000	• FFP dosing = 10–20 mL/kg body weight

TABLE 6–2: Blood Product Common Transfusion Indications

- When transfusing > 1 unit, look for signs of volume overload in patient with premorbid conditions like CHF

- Consider Lasix 20–60 mg IV to prevent volume overload, after each transfusion (e.g., CHF)

PRBC (packed red blood cells), 1 unit → ↑ Hgb by 1 g/dL and Hct by 3–4%

- Acute bleeding with estimated blood loss > 1000 mL or 20% of estimated total blood volume

- Hb ≤ 10 g/dL or Hct ≤ 30% with acute ischemic cardiovascular dz. (angina, MI, CHF)

- Hb ≤ 8.5 g/dL or Hct ≤ 25% in a patient with symptomatic anemia and moderate or major organ dysfunction (NYHA class III/V)

- Hb ≤ 7.5 g/dL or Hct ≤ 23% in a patient with no medical complications (NYHA class I/II)

Autologous red cells

- Hemoglobin ≤ 9 g/dL or hematocrit ≤ 27%

- Surgical blood loss of > 750 mL or 15% of estimated total blood volume

Platelets, 1 apheresis platelet = 6 units of pooled platelets

- Thrombocytopenia < 50,000/µL with active bleeding or prior to procedure

- <15,000/µL in patient who is stable

Note: ITP, TTP, and hemolytic uremic syndrome do not respond to platelet transfusion.

(continued)

TABLE 6–2 (Continued)

Fresh frozen plasma (FFP), dosing: 10–20 mL/kg, 1 unit = 200 mL

- INR > 1.5 and APTT > 50 s with active bleeding

- INR > 1.5 and APTT > 50 s with patient who is undergoing pcinvasive procedure or surgery

- Thrombotic thrombocytopenic purpura (TTP) (FFP that has the cryoprecipitate removed)

- DIC and urgent warfarin reversal

- Liver failure

- Can be useful when specific coagulation factor is not available

Cryoprecipitate, dosing: 1 unit can ↑ fibrinogen by 5–10 mg/dL

- Fibrinogen < 100 mg/dL with active bleeding

- Each concentrate usually contains: factor VIII, VIII + vWF, fibrinogen, XIII

- Indicated in: hemophilia, von Willebrand disease (vWD), DIC

TABLE 6–3: Hypochromic Microcytic Anemia			
	Iron Deficiency	**Thalassemia**	**ACD**
MCHC	↓	↓	N
MCV	↓	↓	N/↓
Iron	↓	N	↓
Ferritin	↓	N	N/↑
TIBC	↑	N	↓
Transferrin saturation	↓	N	N/↑
RDW	↑	N	—
FEP	↑	N	↑
Treatment	Iron sulfate 325 mg tid with orange juice or vitamin C tablets	Confirm thalassemia with Hg electrophoresis	Treat underlying cause

(continued)

TABLE 6–3 (Continued)

Note

- Thalassemia minor: ↓ MCV and basophilic stippling and normal iron, TIBC, transferrin, ferritin, FEP.

- Patient with iron deficiency anemia, retic count should ↑ after 4–6 days after iron supplement.

- Anemia of chronic dz.: can cause either hypochromic microcytic or normochromic normocytic anemia with low retic count.

- If retic count < 2% → bone marrow defect in making RBCs.

- If retic count > 2% → good marrow response to peripheral destruction/hemolysis.

- Reticulocyte index: [retic count % × (patient Hct/normal Hct (45))]

    → If index is 1 → it is considered normal

    → If index is 2–6 → it is considered good marrow response

Abbreviations: MCV, mean corpuscular volume; MCHC, mean corpuscular Hg volume; ACD, anemia of chronic dz.; TIBC, total iron binding capacity; RDW, red cell distribution width; FEP, free erythrocyte protoporphyrin.

TABLE 6–4: Macrocytic Anemia (Megaloblastic Anemia)			
	B_{12} **Deficiency**	**Folate Deficiency**	**Liver Dz.**
MCV	↑	↑	↑
MCHC	N	N	N
Hyper-segmented neutrophil	Present	Present	Not present
Macro-ovalocyte	Present	Present	Not present
Homo-cysteine	↑	↑	NA
Methyl-malonic acid	↑	N	NA
Test	Schilling test		NA
Lab	↓ Cobalamin (B_{12}) (<200 pg/mL)	↓ Serum folate (<2 ng/dL)	LFT, PT, PTT
Rx	Cobalamin 1000 μg (1 mg) IM	Folic acid 1–5 mg/day PO × 4–5 months	Treat underlying cause

(continued)

TABLE 6–4 (Continued)		
Etiologies of Megaloblastic Anemia		
ETOH abuse		Liver disease
Hypothyroidism		Renal disease
Medication Induced		Vegetarians
TMP/SMX	Pyrimethamine	Partial gastrectomy
Methotrexate	OCPs	Pernicious anemia
AZT		Pancreatic insufficiency
		Diphyllobothrium latum

TABLE 6-5: Interpretation of Hemoglobinopathies

Conditions	Hgb A1	Hgb S	Hgb C	Hgb A2	Hgb F
Normal	96–98%			1.5–4%	0–2%
SS disease		60–99%			1–40%
SS trait	60–80%	20–40%			WNL
C disease			95%		5%
Sickle C dz.		45–55%	45–55%		

125

TABLE 6–6: Hemolysis
Leads to
↑ Retic count (>5%)
↓ Hct and haptoglobin
(+) Coombs
↑ Unconjugated bilirubin
↑ LDH, retic count, fragmented RBC
Jaundice

TABLE 6–7: Hypercoagulable Panels	
Antithrombin III	Lupus anticoagulant (antiphospholipid)
PT/PTT	Anticardiolipin (antiphospholipid)
Protein C deficiency	Prothrombin fragment F1.2
Protein S deficiency	Native prothrombin antigen
Factor V Leiden mutation	Heparin neutralization
Antiplasmin	Lipoprotein
Prothrombin mutation 20210A	Plasmin activator inhibitor 1
Plasminogen	Homocysteine level
Cardiovascular risk panel	Phospholipid antibody syndrome/lupus anticoagulant comprehensive panel for
Homocysteine level	• Stroke at young age
Cardio CRP	• DVT
Fibrinogen clotting activity	• Pulmonary HTN
Lipoprotein (a)	• Recurrent miscarriage

(continued)

TABLE 6–7 (Continued)	
Human platelet antigen 1 genotype	Lupus anticoagulant dRVTT confirmation mixing
Soluble P-selectin	Lupus anticoagulant hexagonal phospholipid neut.
von Willebrand Factor antigen	Cardiolipin antibodies, IgA, IgG, and IgM
Factor VII activity	β_2-Glycoprotein I antibodies, IgA, IgG, and IgM
Plasminogen activator inhibitor activity (PAI-1)	Phosphatidylserine antibodies, IgG, and IgM
	Prothrombin antibodies, IgG, and IgM

TABLE 6–8: DVT Prevention

Medical conditions

Heparin 5000 unit Sub Q q12h

Enoxaparin (Lovenox): 40 mg Sub Q once daily;
If CrCl < 30 mL/min ↔ 30 mg Sub Q once daily

Dalteparin (Fragmin): 2500 units Sub Q once daily

Nadroparin[a]: 2850 units Sub Q once daily

General surgery in moderate-risk patient

Heparin 5000 unit Sub Q q12h

Enoxaparin: 20 mg Sub Q 1–2 h before surgery and once daily after surgery

Dalteparin: 2500 units Sub Q 1–2 h before surgery and once daily after surgery

Nadroparin[a]: 2850 units Sub Q 2–4 h before surgery and once daily after surgery

Tinzaparin (Innohep): 3500 units Sub Q 2 h before surgery and once daily after surgery

General surgery in high-risk patient

Heparin 5000 unit Sub Q q8h or q12h

Enoxaparin (Lovenox): 40 mg Sub Q 1–2 h before surgery and once daily after surgery or 30 mg Sub Q every 12 h starting 8–12 h after surgery

Dalteparin (Fragmin): 5000 units Sub Q 8–12 h before surgery and once daily after surgery

(continued)

TABLE 6–8 (Continued)

Orthopedic surgery

Heparin is not recommended

Enoxaparin: 30 mg Sub Q q12h starting 12–24 h after surgery; or 40 mg Sub Q once daily starting 10–12 h postsurgery

Dalteparin: 5000 units Sub Q 8–12 h before surgery, then once daily starting 12–24 h after surgery or 2500 units Sub Q 6–8 h after surgery, then 5000 units Sub Q once daily

Nadroparin[a]: 38 units/kg Sub Q 12 h before surgery, 12 h after surgery, and once daily on postoperative days 1, 2, and 3, then increase to 57 units/kg Sub Q once daily

Tinzaparin: 75 units/kg Sub Q once daily starting 12–24 h after surgery; or 4500 units Sub Q 12 h before surgery and once daily after surgery

Major trauma

Heparin 5000 unit Sub Q q8h

Enoxaparin: 30 mg Sub Q every 12 h
(for acute spinal cord injury)

Enoxaparin: 30 mg Sub Q every 12 h starting 12–36 h after injury if the patient is hemodynamically stable

[a]Not approved.

TABLE 6–9: Guidelines for Management of High INR

- INR above therapeutic and < 5 but no significant bleeding → hold warfarin

- ≥ 5 and <9 and no significant bleeding → hold warfarin

- ≥ 5 and <9 and high risk of bleeding → give vitamin k ≤ 5 mg PO
  - → If rapid reversal needed → 2–4 mg PO and 1–2 mg after 24 h

- >9 and no significant bleeding → hold warfarin and give vitamin K 5–10 mg PO

- Severe bleeding with any INR → hold warfarin and give vitamin K 10 mg IV slow infusion; supplement with FFP or prothrombin complex concentrate (PCC) or recombinant factor VIIa depending on urgency vitamin K 10 mg IV slow infusion can be repeated q12h prn

- Life-threatening bleeding with any INR → hold warfarin and give PCC plus vitamin K 10 mg IV slow. Recombinant factor VIIa can be considered as alternative to PCC

Source with permission: Ansell J, Hirsh J, Poller L, et al. The pharmacology and management of the vitamin K antagonists. *Chest.* 2004;126(3): 204S–233S.

TABLE 6–10: Drugs that Causes Platelet Dysfunction

• Acetazolamide	• Furosemide
• Aminophylline	• Hydralazine
• Amitriptyline	• Hydrocortisone
• Ampicillin	• Hydroxychloroquine
• Aspirin	• Imipramine
• Carbenicillin	• Isoproterenol
• Caffeine	• Lidocaine
• Cephalothin	• Nitroglycerin
• Chlorpromazine	• Nitroprusside
• Cimetidine	• NSAIDs
• Cocaine	• Papaverine
• Colchicine	• Penicillin
• Cyclosporin A	• Promethazine
• Cyproheptadine	• Propranolol
• Diphenhydramine	• Theophylline
• Dipyridamole	• Verapamil
• Ethacrynic acid	• Vinblastine
• Famotidine	• Vincristine

TABLE 6-11: Coagulopathies

↑ PT	↑ PTT	↑ PT and ↑ PTT	↑ Bleeding time
	Inherited		
VII deficiency	vWF deficiency	Prothrombin deficiency	Platelet dysfunction ✗
	VIII deficiency	Fibrinogen deficiency	vWD ↗
	IX deficiency	V deficiency	Paraproteinemia ✗
	XI deficiency	X deficiency	DIC
	XII deficiency		Uremia ↗
			Liver failure
			Factor V deficiency
			Factor VII deficiency
			Factor VIII deficiency
			Factor IX deficiency
	Acquired		
Vitamin K deficiency	Heparin use	Heparin + warfarin	
Warfarin use	Liver dysfunction	Factor II deficiency	
Liver dysfunction	Lupus anticoagulant	Factor V deficiency	

(continued)

TABLE 6–11 (Continued)

Fibrinogen deficiency	Nephrotic syndrome	Factor X deficiency	Factor X deficiency
II deficiency	Hypofibrinogenemia	Liver dz.	Factor XI deficiency
VII deficiency	Antiphospholipid	DIC	Factor XII deficiency
IX deficiency	Factor VIII deficiency	**Vitamin-K-dependent Factors**	
X deficiency	Factor IX deficiency	Factor II	Factor X
V deficiency	Factor XI deficiency	Factor VII	Protein C
Early DIC	Factor XII deficiency	Factor IX	Protein S

Work-up for Abnormal Coagulation Labs

↑ PT and Normal PTT		
D-dimer	LFT	Factor VII level
Fibrinogen	Peripheral smear	

134

↑ PTT and Normal PT		
50:50 mixing study		
→ If PTT corrects, means there is a factor deficiency		
→ If PTT does not correct → check for antiphospholipid antibody and anticardiolipin antibody level		
→ If PTT corrects initially but prolongs on later testing → then check for Factor VIII inhibitor		
↑ PT and ↑ PTT		
	Factor deficiency	
D-dimer	LFT	
Fibrinogen	Peripheral smear	

TABLE 6–12: Management of Bleeding Diathesis

- Treat underlying disorder

- Platelet transfusion: in refractory bleeding (contains: factor VIII, vWF, and fibrinogen)

- Vitamin K: corrects PT/PTT, not useful in acute situtation

- FFP: corrects PT/PTT, useful in acute situation (contains all factors and fibrinogen)

- Cryoprecipitate: raises vWF, useful in DIC to restore fibrinogen level

- Desmopressin: releases stored vWF from cell, prophylaxis before surgery in type I vWD

TABLE 6–13: Tumor Markers

AFP	β Hcg	CA 125
Primary association	**Primary association**	**Primary association**
• Hepatic CA	• Germ cell CA	• Ovarian CA
• Germ cell CA	• Gestational trophoblastic dz.	**Other association**
Other association	**Other association**	• Breast CA
• Biliary CA	• GI CA	• Endometrial CA
• Gastric CA	**BRCA**	• Fallopian tube CA
• Pancreatic CA	**Primary association**	• Esophageal CA
CA 19-9	• Breast cancer	• Gastric CA
Primary association	**Other association**	• Hepatic CA
• Pancreatic CA	• None	• Pancreatic CA
• Biliary tract CA	**PSA**	**CA 153**

(continued)

TABLE 6–13 (Continued)		
Other association	**Primary association**	Mucin breast cancer (MBC)
• Colon CA	• Prostate CA	
• Esophageal CA	**Other association**	
• Hepatic CA	• None	

CA 27.29	CEA
Primary association	**Primary association**
• Breast CA	• Colorectal CA
Other association	**Other association**
• Colon CA	• Bladder CA
• Gastric CA	• Breast CA
• Hepatic CA	• Gastric CA
• Lung CA	• Hepatic CA
• Pancreatic CA	• Medullary CA
• Ovarian CA	• Melanoma
• Prostate CA	• Pancreatic CA

7

Infectious Disease

TABLE 7–1: Note

- When placing patient on an antibiotic consider starting patient on cultured yogurt

- Vancomycin has low lung penetration capacity, use Linezolid

- Calculate creatinine clearance and adjust dose accordingly in renal dysfunction

- Patient with *Staphylococcus aureus* bacteremia → TEE (transesophageal echo) recommended

- CrCl for male (125 mL/min) = (140 – age) × wt (kg)/72 × serum creatinine

- CrCl for female (95 mL/min) = 0.85 × CrCl of male

TABLE 7–2: Antibiotic Properties

	G (+)	G (−)	Atypical	Anaerobe	Pseudomonas	MRSA	MSSA
1st Generation penicillin	+	−	−	−	−	−	−
2nd Generation antistaph PCN	+	−	−	−	−	−	+
3rd Generation amino-PCN	+	±	−	±	−	−	±
4th Generation antipseudomonal PCN	+	+	−	+	+	−	±
1st Generation cephalosporin	+	±	−	−	−	−	+
2nd Generation cephalosporin	+	±	−	±	−	−	+
3rd Generation cephalosporin	±	+	−	±	±	−	±

4th Generation cephalosporin	±	−	+	±	−	±	+
1st Generation quinolones	−	−	−	−	−	+	−
2nd Generation quinolones	−	−	±	−	±	+	−
3rd Generation quinolones	+	−	+	−	+	+	+
4th Generation quinolones	+	−	±	−	+	+	+
Aminoglycoside	+	−	−	−	−	±	−
Macrolide	+	−	−	±	+	±	+
Tetracycline	±	±	−	+	+	±	±

(continued)

143

TABLE 7-2 (Continued)

	G (+)	G (−)	Atypical	Anaerobe	Pseudomonas	MRSA	MSSA
Glycopeptide	+	−	−	±	−	+	+
Carbapenems	+	+	−	+	±	−	+
Ketolide	+	−	−	±	−	−	+
Miscellaneous							
Aztreonam	−	+	−	−	+	−	−
Daptomycin	+	−	−	−	−	+	+
Linezolid	+	±	±	±	−	+	+
Metronidazole	−	−	−	+	−	−	−

TABLE 7-3: Antibiotic Classifications

Penicillins (PCN)

(handwritten: + – Anti Pseud)

1st Generation	2nd Generation	3rd Generation	4th Generation
Benzathine PCN	Dicloxacillin	Amoxicillin	Piperacillin
Bicillin C-R	Nafcillin	Augmentin	Piperacillin–Tazobactam Zosyn
Penicillin G	Oxacillin	Ampicillin	
Penicillin V		Unasyn	Timentin
Procaine PCN		Pivampicillin	

Cephalosporins

(handwritten: + Pseudo)

1st Generation	2nd Generation	3rd Generation	4th Generation
Cefadroxil (Duricef)	Cefaclor (Ceclor)	Cefdinir (Omnicef)	Cefepime (Maxipime)
Cefazolin (Ancef)	Cefotetan	Cefditoren	
Cephalexin (Keflex)	Cefoxitin	Cefixime (Suprax)	

(continued)

145

TABLE 7-3 (Continued)

Cephalosporins

	Cefprozil	Cefoperazone
	Cefuroxime	Claforan
	Lorabid	Cefpodoxime
		Ceftazidime (Fortaz)
		Ceftizoxime
		Ceftriaxone (Rocephin)

Quinolones

1st Generation	2nd Generation	3rd Generation — + Atyp *(Pseudo)*	4th Generation — + Atyp
Nalidixic acid (NegGram)	Ciprofloxacin	Levofloxacin (Levaquin)	Gatifloxacin (Tequin)
	Enoxacin		
	Lomefloxacin		Gemifloxacin

Norfloxacin		Moxifloxacin (Avelox)
Ofloxacin		

Aminoglycosides	**Macrolides**
Amikacin	Azithromycin (Zithromax)
Gentamicin	Clarithromycin (Biaxin)
Streptomycin	Dirithromycin (Dynabac)
Tobramycin	Erythromycin
Carbapenems	**Tetracyclines**
Ertapenem (Invanz)	Doxycycline (Adoxa, Doryx, Monodox)
Imipenem–cilastatin (Primaxin)	Minocycline
Meropenem (Merrem)	Tetracycline
Glycopeptide	**Ketolide**
Vancomycin	Telithromycin (Ketek)

TABLE 7–4: Medication—Peak and Trough Levels

Medication	Peak	Trough
Amikacin	Peak 20–30 μg/mL	<10 μg/mL
Gentamicin (Garamycin)	6–8 μg/mL	<2 μg/mL
Streptomycin	15–40 μg/mL	<5 μg/mL
Vancomycin (Vancocin)	20–40 μg/mL (usually not performed)	5–15 μg/mL (cellulitis)
		10–20 μg/mL (pneumonia/endocarditis)
Note		

- Check vancomycin trough level before 3rd or 4th dose.
- Check gentamicin trough level before 4th dose.
- Amikacin: obtain peak level 30 min after a 30 min infusion; obtain trough level within 30 min prior to next dose.

TABLE 7–5: Aspergillosis

- Amphotericin B deoxycholate 1–1.5 mg/kg IV daily × 2 weeks 1st line

- Voriconazole 6 mg/kg IV bid × 1 day then 4 mg/kg/12 h × 2 weeks 1st line

- Caspofungin 70 mg IV × 1 dose then 50 mg IV daily × 2 weeks 2nd line

- Itraconazole 200 mg IV q12h × 2 days then 200 mg IV daily × 2 weeks 2nd line

- Abelcet 5 mg/kg/day IV × 2 weeks 2nd line

TABLE 7–6: *Candida* in Blood

- *C. albicans, C. tropicalis, C. parapsilosis*

- Fluconazole 800 mg IV × 1 dose then 400 mg IV daily × 2 week 1st line

- Caspofungin (Cancidas) 70 mg IV × 1 dose then 50 mg IV daily × 2 weeks 1st line

- Amphotericin B deoxycholate 0.7 mg/kg IV daily × 2 weeks 1st line

- Abelcet 5 mg/kg/day IV × 2 weeks 2nd line

- Itraconazole 200 mg IV q12h × 2 days then 200 mg IV daily × 2 weeks 2nd line

- *C. glabrata, C. krusei*

- Caspofungin (Cancidas) 70 mg IV × 1 dose then 50 mg IV daily × 2 weeks

TABLE 7–7: Cellulitis

- Cefazolin 1 g IV q6-8h 1st line
- Nafcillin 1–1.5 g IV q4-6h 1st line
- Ceftriaxone 1 g IV q24h 1st line
- Cefazolin 2 g IV q24h + probenecid 1 g PO daily 1st line

If MRSA or penicillin allergy

- Vancomycin 1–2 g IV daily 1st line
- Linezolid 0.6 g IV q12h 1st line

Note: Patient can be switched to oral medication once patient is afebrile and resolution of cellulitis is noted.

- Dicloxacillin 0.5 g PO q6h 1st line
- Cephradine 0.5 g PO q6h 1st line
- Cephalexin 0.5 g PO q6h 1st line
- Cefadroxil 0.5–1 g PO q12-24h 1st line

Cellulitis associated with specific condition

- Penicillin allergy: erythromycin 500 mg PO q6h
- Human bite: amoxicillin–clavulanate (Augmentin) or cefoxitin IV
- Animal bite: penicillin IV or nafcillin IV or cefoxitin IV
- Facial cellulitis: cefotaxime IV, if oral cavity involved cover anaerobes with clindamycin/flagyl
- Diabetic patient: cefoxitin or clindamycin + gentamicin
- IV drug abuse: vancomycin + gentamicin

TABLE 7–7 (Continued)
• Burn patient: vancomycin + gentamicin
• Compromised patient: clindamycin + gentamicin
• Suspicion of anaerobe: clindamycin 600 mg IV q8h or metronidazole 500 mg IV q6h
• Gas forming infection: clindamycin 600 mg IV q8h or metronidazole 500 mg IV q6h
Source with permission: Morton N. Swartz, MD.Cellulitis, *N Engl J Med.* 2004;350:9.

TABLE 7–8: Cholecystitis/Cholangitis
• Ampicillin + gentamicin (adjust for renal dose) 1st line
• Piperacillin–tazobactam (Zosyn) 3.375 g q6h IV 1st line
• Ampicillin–sulbactam (Unasyn) 3 g q6h IV 1st line
• Ticarcillin–clavulanate (Timentin) 3.1 g q6h IV 1st line
• 3rd Generation cephalosporin + metronidazole 500 mg PO qid or 15 mg/kg IV q12h 2nd line
• Aztreonam 2 g IV q8h + metronidazole 500 mg PO qid or 15 mg/kg IV q12h 2nd line
• Ciprofloxacin 400 mg IV q12h + metronidazole 500 mg PO qid or 15 mg/kg IV q12h 2nd line

TABLE 7–9: *Clostridium difficile* Infection

- Metronidazole 500 mg PO tid or 250 mg PO/IV qid × 10–14 days 1st line

- Vancomycin 125 mg PO qid × 10–14 days (IV is not effective) 2nd line

- Bacitracin 25,000 units PO qid × 10–14 days 3rd line

- Cholestyramine 4 g PO tid × 10–14 days (use in addition to above Abx, for relapsing *C. difficile*)

Note: Add Florastor 250 mg 1 tab PO bid for recurrent *C. difficile*.

TABLE 7–10: Conjunctivitis (Non–specific)

- Get ophthalmology consult prior to starting patient on steroid ophthalmic drops

- Erythromycin ophthalmic ointment $1/2$ in. qid for 5–7 days or

- Sulfacetamide ophthalmic drops 10% 1–2 gtts (drop) in each eye q6-8h for 5–7 days

- Eye lubricant drops → Hypotears/Refresh/Tears II 1–2 drops q1h qid prn

- Eye lubricant ointment → Lacrilube/Refresh PM $1/2$ in. qhs or qid prn

TABLE 7–11: Conjunctivitis (Bacterial)

- Polytrim ophthalmic solution 1–2 gtts (drop) in each eye q3-6h for 5–7 days or

- Erythromycin ophthalmic ointment $1/2$ in. qid for 5–7 days or

- Sulfacetamide ophthalmic drops 10% 1–2 gtts (drop) in each eye q6-8h for 5–7 days or

- Quinolone ophthalmic drops (Ciloxan, Ocuflox) 1–2 gtts in each eye q6-8h × 5–7 days or

- Ofloxacin 1–2 gtts (drops) in each eye q2h for 1–2 days or qid 3–7 days or

- Ciprofloxacin 1–2 gtts (drops) in each eye q2h for 1–2 days or qid 3–7 days or

- Levofloxacin 1–2 gtts (drops) in each eye q2h for 1–2 days or qid 3–7 days or

- Bacitracin ophthalmic ointment $1/4 - 1/2$ in. q4h for 7 days or

- Tobrex solution 1–2 gtts q4h

TABLE 7–12: Conjunctivitis (Viral)

- Naphcon-A 1–2 drops qid for symptomatic relief (do not use > 3 weeks) or

- Ocuhist 1–2 drops qid for symptomatic relief (do not use > 3 weeks) or

- Visine AC 1–2 drops qid for symptomatic relief (do not use > 3 weeks)

TABLE 7–13: Conjunctivitis (Allergic)

• 1st line → Naphcon-A 1–2 drops qid for symptomatic relief (do not use > 3 weeks) or
→ Ocuhist 1–2 drops qid for symptomatic relief (do not use > 3 weeks)
→ Visine AC 1–2 drops qid for symptomatic relief (do not use > 3 weeks)
• 2nd line → Patanol 1–2 drops bid or
→ Acular 1–2 drops qid
• 3rd line → use in conjunction with 1st and 2nd line Rx
→ Alomide 1–2 drops qid or
→ Opticrom 1–2 drops qid or
→ Crolom 1–2 drops qid

TABLE 7–14: Diverticulitis

- Consider placing patient NPO/clear liquid

Mild diverticulitis (treat for 7–10 days)

- TMP–SMX DS PO bid 1st line

- Ciprofloxacin 750 mg PO bid 1st line

- Levofloxacin 750 mg PO daily + metronidazole 500 mg PO q6h 1st line

- Amoxicillin/clavulanate ER 1000/62.5 mg 2 tab PO bid 2nd line

Mild–moderate

- Zosyn (piperacillin + tazobactam) 3.375 g IV q6h or 4.5 g IV q8h 1st line

- Unasyn (ampicillin + sulbactam) 3 g IV q6h 1st line

- Timentin (ticarcillin + clavulanate) 3.1 g IV q6h 1st line

- Ertapenem 1 g IV daily 1st line

- Ciprofloxacin 400 mg IV q12h 2nd line

- Levofloxacin 750 mg IV q24h + metronidazole 500 mg IV q6h 2nd line

(continued)

TABLE 7–14 (Continued)
Severe
→ Imipenem–cilastatin (Primaxin) 500 mg IV q6h 1st line
→ Meropenem 1 g IV q8h 1st line
→ Ampicillin 2 g IV q6h + metronidazole 500 mg IV q6h + ciprofloxacin 400 mg IV q12h 2nd line
→ Ampicillin 2 g IV q6h + metronidazole 500 mg IV q6h + levofloxacin 750 mg IV q24h 2nd line
→ Ampicillin 2 g IV q6h + metronidazole 500 mg IV q6h + (gentamicin or amikacin) 2nd line

TABLE 7–15: Duke Criteria for Infective Endocarditis (IE)

- Two major criteria or 1 major and 3 minor criteria or 5 minor criteria

Major Criteria	Minor Criteria
1. (+) Blood culture	**1. Fever ≥ 38°C (100.4°F)**
A. Atypical organisms associated with IE	**2. Hx of heart condition or IV drug use**
• *S. viridans, S. bovis*	**3. Microbiological evidence**
• HACEK[a]	A. (+) Blood Cx but does not meet Major criteria or
	B. Serological evidence of active evidence with organism consistent with IE
2. Persistently positive blood cultures	
A. Defined as 2(+) blood cultures > 12 h apart	**4. Vascular phenomenon**
B. All 3 or a majority of 4 cultures (1st and 4th 1 h apart)	A. Major arterial emboli
	B. Septic pulmonary infarct

(continued)

TABLE 7–15 (Continued)	
3. (+) Echocardiogram	C. Mycotic aneurysm
A. Oscillating intracardial mass on valve or supporting structure	D. Conjunctival/ intracranial hemorrhage
	E. Janeway lesion
B. Abscess	**5. Immunologic phenomenon**
C. New partial dehiscence of prosthetic valve	A. Glomerulonephritis
4. New murmur	B. Osler's node
	C. Roth spots
	D. Rheumatoid factor
	6. Echocardiographic finding
	That does not meet major criteria
[a]HACEK: *Haemophilus, Actinobacillus, Cardiobacterium hominis, Eikenella corrodens, Kingella.*	

TABLE 7–16: Von Reyn Criteria for Diagnosis of Infective Endocarditis (IE)

- **Definite infective endocarditis**

1. Direct evidence by histology, bacteriology, valvular vegetation or peripheral emboli

- **Probable infective endocarditis**

1. Persistently (+) blood Cx + 1 of the following

   A. New regurgitant murmur

   B. Predisposing heart disease or vascular phenomenon

2. Negative or intermittently positive blood cultures + 3 of the following

   A. Fever

   B. New regurgitant murmur

   C. Vascular phenomenon (i.e., splinter/conjunctival hemorrhage, petechiae, Roth spots, emboli)

- **Possible infective endocarditis**

1. Persistently (+) blood Cx + 1 of the following

   A. Predisposing heart disease (exclude permanent heart disease)

   B. Vascular phenomenon

2. Negative or intermittently positive blood cultures + 3 of the following

   A. Predisposing heart disease

   B. Vascular phenomenon

   C. Fever

TABLE 7-17: Endocarditis Prophylaxis[a]

Dental Procedures

• Dental extraction	• Endodontic instrumentation
• Periodontal procedure	• Dental implant placement
• Prophylactic cleaning of teeth of implants where bleeding is anticipated	• Initial placement of orthodontic band

Respiratory Tract

• Tonsillectomy	• Adenoidectomy
• Bronchoscopy with a rigid bronchoscope	• Procedure that involves respiratory mucosa

Prophylaxis for Dental and Respiratory Tract Procedure

PO → Amoxicillin 2 g PO; children 50 mg/kg PO 1 h prior to procedure

→ PCN allergy → clindamycin 600 mg PO; children 20 mg/kg PO 1 h prior to procedure or

→ Azithromycin or clarithromycin 500 mg; children 15 mg/kg PO 1 h prior to procedure or

→ Cephalexin or cefadroxil 2 g; children 50 mg/kg PO 1 h prior to procedure

Parenteral → Ampicillin 2 g IM/IV; children 50 mg/kg IM/IV 30 min before the procedure or

→ Clindamycin 600 mg IV; children 20 mg/kg IV 30 min before the procedure or

→ Cefazolin 1 g IV; children 25 mg/kg IM/IV 30 min before the procedure

TABLE 7–17 (Continued)

Gastrointestinal Tract

• Sclerotherapy for esophageal varices	• Esophageal stricture dilation
• ERCP	• Biliary tract surgery
• Surgical procedure that involves intestinal mucosa	

Prophylaxis for Gastrointestinal Procedure

PO → Amoxicillin 2 g PO; children 50 mg/kg PO 1 h before or

→ Ampicillin 2 g IM/IV; children 50 mg/kg IM/IV within 30 min of starting the procedure

→ PCN allergy →vancomycin 1 g over 1–2 h (children 20 mg/kg IV over 1–2 h), complete infusion within 30 min of starting the procedure

Parenteral → Ampicillin 2 g IM/IV (children 50 mg/kg IM/IV) + gentamicin 1.5 mg/kg IM/IV within 30 min of starting the procedure;

→ PCN tballergy → vancomycin 1 g IV (children 20 mg/kg IV) slowly over 1–2 h + gentamicin 1.5 mg/kg IM/IV 30 min of starting the procedure

Genitourinary Tract

• Prostatic surgery	• Cystoscopy/urethral dilation

(continued)

TABLE 7–17 (Continued)

Prophylaxis for Genitourinary Procedure

PO → Amoxicillin 2 g PO; children 50 mg/kg PO 1 h before or

→ Ampicillin 2 g IM/IV; children 50 mg/kg IM/IV within 30 min of starting the procedure

→ PCN allergy → Vancomycin 1 g (children 20 mg/kg IV over 1–2 h) over 1–2 h, complete infusion within 30 min of starting the procedure

Parenteral → Ampicillin 2 g IM/IV (children 50 mg/kg IM/IV) + gentamicin 1.5 mg/kg IM/IV within 30 min of starting the procedure

→ PCN allergy → vancomycin 1 g IV slowly over 1–2 h (children 20 mg/kg IV over 1–2 h) + gentamicin 1.5 mg/kg IM/IV 30 min of starting the procedure

Endocarditis

- Streptococci[b]: penicillin 2–4 million units IV q4h + gentamicin × 2 weeks

Note: Use only penicillin × 4 weeks in patient with renal insufficiency or cranial N8 damage.

- Enterococci[b]: penicillin 5–10 million units IV q4h + (gentamicin/streptomycin)× 4–6 weeks

- *Staphylococcus* (native valve): oxacillin or nafcillin 2 g IV q4h × 6 weeks (use gentamicin for initial 3–5 days)

- *Staphylococcus* (prosthetic valve): vancomycin 15 mg/kg IV infused over 1 h q12h × 6 weeks + rifampin 300 mg PO q8h × 6 weeks + gentamicin for 1st 2 weeks

- HACEK organisms: ceftriaxone 2 g IV/IM q24h × 4 weeks

TABLE 7–17 (Continued)

If Penicillin Allergy

Penicillin susceptible streptococci

- Vancomycin[c] 15 mg/kg IV over 1 h q12h + gentamicin for 4–6 h

- Ceftriaxone 2 g IV IM × 4 weeks or

- Ceftriaxone 2 g IV + gentamicin 3 mg/kg daily × 2 weeks

Note: Prosthetic valve endocarditis: treat for 6 weeks.

Enterococci

- Consider penicillin desensitization

- Vancomycin[c] 15 mg/kg IV over 1 h q12h + gentamicin × 4–6 weeks

Note: Prosthetic valve endocarditis: treat for 6 weeks.

***Staphylococcus* (native valve)**

- Cefazolin[d] 2 g IV q8h

- Vancomycin[c] 15 mg/kg IV over 1 h q12h × 6 weeks

[a]Endocarditis prophylaxis is recommended for patient with high and moderate risk cardiac disease.
[b]Patient with prosthetic valve treat for 6 weeks.
[c]Vancomycin usual dose 1 g over 1 h q12h.
[d]Consider not using in patient with type I hypersensitivity.

Source with permission: Dajani AS, Taubert KA, Wilson W, et al. Prevention of bacterial endocarditis: Antibiotic prophylaxis. *JAMA* 1997;277:1797.

TABLE 7–18: HIV Opportunistic Infection

Aspergillosis

Voriconazole 6 mg/kg IV q12h × 1 day then 4 mg/kg IV q12h 1st line

Amphotericin B 0.7–1.4 mg/kg daily 2nd line

Caspofungin 70 mg IV daily then 50 mg IV daily 2nd line

Bartonella henselae and *quintana*

Erythromycin 500 mg PO qid 1st line

Doxycycline 100 mg PO bid 2nd line

Azithromycin 0.5–1 g PO daily 2nd line

Doxycycline 100 mg PO bid + rifampin 300 mg IV/PO bid

Candida spp.

Esophagitis

Fluconazole 200 mg PO daily 1st line

Itraconazole 200 mg PO daily (take on an empty stomach) 2nd line

Voriconazole 200 mg PO bid

Caspofungin 70 mg IV q24h × 1 day then 50 mg IV q24h

Thrush

Clotrimazole oral troches 10 mg 5 × a day 1st line

Nystatin 500,000 units gargle 4–5 times a day 2nd line

Fluconazole 100 mg PO daily 2nd line

Itraconazole 100 mg oral suspension swish and swallow daily 2nd line

TABLE 7–18 (Continued)
Amphotericin B 0.3–0.5 mg/kg IV daily 2nd line
Vaginitis
Butoconazole 2% cream apply daily 1st line
Clotrimazole 1% cream apply daily 1st line
Miconazole 2% cream day or 100 mg vaginal supp apply daily 1st line
Ketoconazole 200 mg PO bid
Coccidioides immitis (**Coccidiomycosis**)
Pulmonary or disseminated
Amphotericin B 0.5–1 mg/kg IV q24h ± fluconazole
Meningitis
Fluconazole 400–800 mg PO daily 1st line
Itraconazole 200–400 mg PO bid 2nd line
Cryptococcus neoformans
Meningitis
Amphotericin B 0.7 mg/kg IV daily + 5 FC 100 mg/kg PO daily 1st line
Fluconazole 400–800 mg PO daily + 5 FC 100 mg/kg PO daily 2nd line
AmBisome 4 mg/kg IV daily 2nd line
Pulmonary or disseminated
Fluconazole 200–400 mg PO daily 1st line
Itraconazole 200 mg PO bid (take on an empty stomach) 2nd line

(continued)

TABLE 7–18 (Continued)
Cryptosporidium parvum
HAART (highly active antiretroviral therapy) 1st line
Nitazoxanide 500 mg PO bid 3rd line
Paromomycin 1 g PO bid + azithromycin 600 mg PO daily 3rd line
Atovaquone 750 mg suspension PO bid with meal 3rd line
Cytomegalovirus (CMV)
Retinitis
Ganciclovir implant q6 months + valganciclovir 900 mg PO bid 1st line
Ganciclovir 5 mg/kg IV bid 1st line
Foscarnet 60 mg/kg IV q8h or 90 mg/kg q12h 1st line
Valganciclovir 900 mg PO bid
Cidofovir 5 mg/kg IV twice a week + probenecid 2 g PO q3h 2nd line
Extraocular disease (GI: esophagitis or colitis)
Valganciclovir 900 mg PO bid 1st line
Ganciclovir 5 mg/kg IV bid 1st line
Foscarnet 60 mg/kg q8h or 90 mg/kg IV q12h 1st line
Neurological disease
Ganciclovir 5 mg/kg IV bid + foscarnet 90 mg/kg IV bid 1st line
Ganciclovir 5 mg/kg IV bid 2nd line

TABLE 7–18 (Continued)

Pneumonitis

Ganciclovir 5 mg/kg IV bid 1st line

Foscarnet 60 mg/kg q8h or 90 mg/kg IV q12h 1st line

Valganciclovir 900 mg PO bid 1st line

Entamoeba histolytica

Metronidazole 750 mg IV/PO tid + diiodohydroxyquin 650 mg PO tid + paromomycin 500 mg PO tid 1st line

Paromomycin 500 mg PO tid 2nd line

Haemophilus influenzae

Cefuroxime 1st line

TMP–SMX 2nd line

2nd or 3rd generation cephalosporin 2nd line

Fluoroquinolones 2nd line

Herpes Simplex

Labialis

Acyclovir 400 mg PO tid, severe: 5–10 mg/kg IV q8h 1st line

Famciclovir 500 mg PO bid 1st line

Valacyclovir 1 g PO bid 1st line

Penciclovir topical q2h (use in conjunction with valacyclovir, famciclovir, or acyclovir) 1st line

Pneumonitis, esophagitis, hepatitis, or dissemination

Acyclovir 5–10 mg/kg IV q8h

(continued)

TABLE 7–18 (Continued)

Encephalitis

Acyclovir 10 mg/kg IV q8h

Herpes Zoster

Dermatomal

Famciclovir 500 mg PO tid 1st line

Valacyclovir 1 g PO tid 1st line

Acyclovir 30 mg/kg IV daily 1st line for severe disease

Ophthalmic or visceral involvement

Acyclovir 30–36 mg/kg IV daily for 1st line

Foscarnet 40 mg/kg IV q8h or 60 mg/kg q12h 2nd line

Chickenpox

Acyclovir 10 mg/kg IV q8h or 800 mg PO qid 1st line

Valacyclovir 1 g q8h 2nd line

Histoplasma capsulatum

Amphotericin B 0.7 mg/kg IV daily 1st line

AmBisome 3–5 mg/kg IV daily 1st line

Fluconazole 800 mg PO daily 2nd line

Isospora belli (Isosporiasis)

TMP–SMX two DS PO bid or one DS tid 1st line

Pyrimethamine 50–75 mg PO daily + leucovorin acid 5–10 mg PO daily

TABLE 7–18 (Continued)

JC virus (progressive multifocal leukoencephalopathy)

HAART 1st line

Interferon alpha 3 MU daily 2nd line

Cidofovir + HAART 2nd line

Microsporidia (microsporidiosis)

E. bieneusi: fumagillin 60 mg PO daily (may cause neutropenia and thrombocytopenia) 1st line

E. intestinalis: albendazole 400 mg PO bid 1st line

Ocular: Fumidil B 3 mg/mL saline eye drops 1st line

Metronidazole 500 mg PO tid 2nd line

Nitazoxanide 500 mg PO bid (currently in an experimental stage) 3rd line

Mycobacterium avium complex (MAC)

Clarithromycin 500 mg PO bid + ethambutol 15 mg/kg PO daily 1st line

Azithromycin 500–600 mg PO daily + ethambutol 15 mg/kg PO daily 1st line

Severe symptoms: above two drugs + ciprofloxacin 500–750 mg PO bid 1st line

Above two drugs + levofloxacin 500–750 mg PO daily 1st line

Above two drugs + rifabutin 300 mg PO daily 1st line

(continued)

TABLE 7–18 (Continued)

Mycobacterium chelonae

Clarithromycin 500 mg PO bid 1st line

Cefoxitin or amikacin or doxycycline or imipenem or erythromycin or tobramycin 2nd line

Mycobacterium fortuitum

Amikacin 400 mg IV q12h + cefoxitin 1–2 g IV daily

Mycobacterium kansasii

INH 300 mg PO daily + rifampin 600 mg PO daily + EMB 25 mg/kg daily ± streptomycin 1 g IM

Ciprofloxacin 750 mg PO bid + clarithromycin 500 mg PO bid

Mycobacterium scrofulaceum

Surgical excision 1st line

Mycobacterium tuberculosis

INH + rifampin + PZA + EMB × 8 weeks then INH + rifampin × 18 weeks 1st line

INH + rifabutin + PZA + EMB × 8 weeks then INH + rifabutin × 18 weeks 2nd line

Latent TB

INH 300 mg PO daily + pyridoxine 50 mg PO daily 1st line

INH 900 mg PO twice a week + pyridoxine 50 mg PO twice a week 1st line

TABLE 7–18 (Continued)

Nocardia asteroides

Trisulfapyridine 3–12 g PO daily 1st line

TMP–SMX 5–15 mg/kg PO daily 1st line

Minocycline 100 mg PO bid 2nd line

Penicillium marneffei

Amphotericin B 0.7–1 mg/kg IV daily 1st line

Itraconazole 200 mg PO bid

Pneumocystis carinii (PCP)

Trimethoprim 15 mg/kg PO daily + sulfamethoxazole 75 mg/kg PO/IV daily 1st line

Hypoxemia: add prednisone 40 mg PO bid

TMP 15 mg/kg PO daily + dapsone 100 mg PO daily 2nd line

Pentamidine 3–4 mg/kg IV q24h 2nd line

Clindamycin 600–900 mg IV q6-8h + primaquine 15–30 mg PO daily 2nd line

Atovaquone 750 mg suspension PO bid 2nd line

Pseudomonas aeruginosa

Aminoglycoside + antipseudomonal β-lactam 1st line

Antipseudomonal β-lactam 2nd line

Carbapenem 2nd line

Ciprofloxacin 2nd line

Aminoglycoside 2nd line

(continued)

TABLE 7–18 (Continued)

Salmonella spp.

Ciprofloxacin 500 mg PO bid 1st line

TMP 1 DS PO bid 2nd line

Staphylococcus aureus

MSSA: nafcillin or oxacillin ± gentamicin 1 mg/kg IV q8h 1st line

Cephalexin 500 mg PO qid 1st line

Dicloxacillin 500 mg PO qid 1st line

Clindamycin 300 mg PO tid 1st line

Fluoroquinolone 1st line

First generation cephalosporin ± gentamicin or rifampin 2nd line

MRSA: Vancomycin 1 g IV q12h ± gentamicin or rifampin 1st line

Linezolid 600 mg PO/IV bid

Streptococcus pneumoniae

Penicillin or amoxicillin or cefotaxime, ceftriaxone or fluoroquinolone 1st line

Macrolide or vancomycin 2nd line

TABLE 7–18 (Continued)

Toxoplasma gondii

Pyrimethamine 200 mg PO loading dose then 50–75 mg PO daily + leucovorin 10–20 mg PO daily + sulfadiazine 1–1.5 g PO q6h 1st line

Pyrimethamine + leucovorin + clindamycin 600 mg IV q6h 2nd line

TMP 5 mg/kg PO bid + SMX 25 mg/kg PO bid 2nd line

5 Fluorouracil 1.5 mg/kg PO daily + clindamycin 1.8–2.4 g PO/IV bid 2nd line

Treponema pallidum (Syphilis)

Primary, secondary, and early latent syphilis (<1 year)

Benzathine penicillin G 2.4 million units IM × 1 dose

Primary, secondary, and early latent syphilis (>1 year or unknown)

Benzathine penicillin G 2.4 million units IM weekly × 3 weeks

Neurosyphilis

Aqueous penicillin G 18–24 million units IV daily × 10–14 days

Source with permission: Bartlett J, Gallant J. Medical Management of HIV Infection. Baltimore, MD: Johns Hopkins University, 2003.

TABLE 7–19: Meningitis

Signs and Symptoms		
• Fever	• Stiff neck	• Rash
• Headache	• Photophobia	• Rhinorrhea
• Cough	• Earache	• Otorrhea
• Brudzinski's sign: bending chin to chest can cause hips and knees flex		
• Kernig's sign: straight leg raising can cause pain		
Tests		
• CT with contrast	• Lumbar puncture	• CBC
• Blood culture	• CXR	• HIV
• If nasal discharge → test for: glucose and chloride to R/O CSF leak		
Therapy		
• Antibiotic should be given empirically before if there is high suspicion of meningitis		
• LP can be done within 2 h after first dose of empiric antibiotic Rx		
• Steroids IV to reduce cerebral edema; dexamethasone 0.15 mg/kg IV bolus then 4 mg IV q6h		

TABLE 7–19 (Continued)

Bacterial Meningitis Empiric Treatment

Preterm and low weight neonate	Group B Strep, *L. monocytogenes*, *E. coli*, Staphylococci, G (–)	Vancomycin (Vanco) 15 mg/kg IV q6h + ceftazidime 50–100 mg/kg q8h
0–3 months	Group B Strep, *L. monocytogenes*, *E. coli*	Ampicillin 50 mg/kg IV q8h + ceftriaxone 50–100 mg/kg IV q12h
3 months–18 years	*S. pneumoniae*, *H. influenzae*, *N. meningitis*	Ceftriaxone 50–100 mg/kg IV q12h + Vanco 10 mg/kg IV q6h
18 years–50 years immunocompetent	*S. pneumoniae*, *N. meningitis*	Ceftriaxone 2 g IV q12h + Vanco 500 mg IV q6h
>50 years immunocompetent	*N. meningitis*, *L. monocytogenes*, G (–) bacilli	Ampicillin 2 g IV q4h + ceftriaxone 2 g IV q2h + Vanco 500 mg IV q6h

(continued)

TABLE 7–19 (Continued)		
Immuno-compromised	*L. monocytogenes*, G (–) bacilli	Ampicillin 2 g IV q4h + ceftazidime 50–100 mg/kg IV q8h
Head trauma, shunt, or surgery	Staphylococci, G (–) bacilli, *S. pneumoniae*	Vanco 15 mg/kg IV q6h + ceftazidime 50–100 mg/kg IV q8h

Source with permission: Quagliarello VJ, Sheld WM. Treatment of bacterial meningitis. *N Engl J Med*. 1997;336:708.

TABLE 7–20: Meningococcal Infection: Chemoprophylaxis

Age	Medication
<1 month	Rifampin 5 mg/kg PO q12h × 2 days
>1 month	Rifampin 20 mg/kg PO q12h × 2 days
<12 years	Ceftriaxone 125 mg IM × 1 dose
>12 years	Ceftriaxone 250 mg IM × 1 dose
Adult	Rifampin 600 mg/kg PO q12h × 2 days or ciprofloxacin 500 mg PO × 1 dose

Note

Rifampin

- Not recommended for pregnant female, it may reduce reliability of oral contraceptive pills.

- It may cause red-orange discoloration of body fluids (urine, tears, and so on).

Ciprofloxacin

- Not recommended if < 18 years of age, pregnant female, or lactating female.

- It can be used in children if no other alternative is available.

Source with permission: Meningococcal disease: evaluation and management of suspected outbreaks, MMWR, Morbidity Mortality Weekly Report. 1997;46(RR-6):6.

TABLE 7–21: MRSA (Methicillin-resistant *staph aureus*)

- Vancomycin 1 g IV q12h (it has poor lung penetration) 1st line

- TMP–SMX DS 1 tab PO bid 1st line

- Dicloxacillin 500 mg PO qid 1st line

- Linezolid (Zyvox) 600 mg IV/PO bid (SE: thrombocytopenia) 2nd line

- Daptomycin (Cubicin) → CrCl ≥ 30 → 4 mg/kg/day, <30 → 4 mg/kg every other day 2nd line

- Clindamycin 300–450 mg PO tid 2nd line

- Fluoroquinolones (ciprofloxacin, moxifloxacin, and levofloxacin) 2nd line

- Tigecycline (Tygacil) 2nd line

Note: Patient with *S. aureus* bacteremia → TEE recommended.

TABLE 7–22: MSSA (Methicillin-sensitive *staph aureus*)

- Nafcillin 2 g q4h IV × 4–6 weeks 1st line

- Cefazolin 2 g IV q8h (Ancef) 1st line

- Vancomycin 1 g IV q12h (it has poor lung penetration) 2nd line

Note: Patient with *S. aureus* bacteremia → TEE recommended.

TABLE 7–23: Osteomyelitis

- Nafcillin/oxacillin 2 g IV q4h 1st line

- Ancef 1–2 g IV q8h 1st line

- Unasyn (ampicillin + sulbactam) 1.5–3 g IV q6h 1st line

- Zosyn 3.375–4.5 g IV q6h 2nd line

- Linezolid (Zyvox) 600 mg IV/PO q12h 2nd line
  (SE: thrombocytopenia)

- MRSA suspected or penicillin allergy: vancomycin
  1 g IV q12h

- Anaerobe suspected: clindamycin 600 mg IV q6h

- Aerobes and anaerobe suspected: clindamycin + 3rd
  generation cephalosporin or quinolone

- Diabetic or bite wound: clindamycin + 3rd generation
  cephalosporin or quinolone

- Hyperbaric oxygen (not proven by randomized controlled
  studies)

TABLE 7–24: Pelvic Inflammatory Disease/ Salpingitis/Tuboovarian Abscess

- Doxycycline 200 mg IV q12h × 3 days then 100 mg IV q12h × 11 days + cefoxitin 2 g IV q6h × 2 weeks or cefotetan 2 g IV q12h × 2 weeks or ertapenem 1 g IV q24h × 3–10 days 1st line

- Doxycycline 200 mg IV q12h × 3 days then 100 mg IV q12h × 11 days + ampicillin/sulbactam 3 g IV q6h × 2 weeks 2nd line

- Ciprofloxacin 400 mg IV/500 mg PO q12h + metronidazole 1 g IV q24h × 2 weeks 2nd line

- Gatifloxacin 400 mg IV/PO q24h + metronidazole 1 g IV q24h × 2 weeks 2nd line

- Levofloxacin 500 mg IV/PO q24h + metronidazole 1 g IV q24h × 2 weeks 2nd line

- Moxifloxacin 400 mg IV/PO q24h + metronidazole 1 g IV q24h × 2 weeks 2nd line

- Ofloxacin 400 mg IV/PO q12h + metronidazole 1 g IV q24h × 2 weeks 2nd line

TABLE 7–25: Peritonitis (Bacterial)

Mild–moderate
(2° from appendicitis, diverticulitis, and so on)

- Ceftriaxone 1–2 g IV q24h + metronidazole 1 g IV q24h 1st line

- Moxifloxacin 400 mg IV q24h or Unasyn 1.5 g q6h or ceftizoxime 2 g IV q8h or cefoxitin 2 g IV q6h 2nd line

Severe peritonitis
(2° from appendicitis, diverticulitis, and so on)

- Meropenem 1 g IV q8h 1st line

- Piperacillin/tazobactam 4.5 g IV q8h 1st line

- Ertapenem 1 g IV q24h 1st line

- Imipenem 500 mg IV q6h 1st line

Spontaneous bacterial peritonitis

- Ceftriaxone 1 g IV q24h 1st line

- Ciprofloxacin 400 mg IV or 500 mg PO q12h 1st line

- Gatifloxacin 400 mg IV/PO q24h 1st line

- Levofloxacin 500 mg IV/PO q24h 1st line

- Moxifloxacin 400 mg IV/PO q24h 1st line

- Aztreonam 2 g IV q8h 2nd line

TABLE 7–26: PORT Criteria (Pneumonia Assessment Scale [PAS])

- If patient's age is ≥ 50 years → go to risk factor table and assign patient in class II–V

- If < 50 years then assign class I to this individual

- If < 50 years and has any of the following conditions or physical examination abnormalities then → go to risk factor table and assign patient in class II–V, otherwise assign class I to this individual

Conditions	Physical Examination Abnormality	
• Active neoplastic dz.	• Altered mental status	
• Congestive heart failure	• Pulse ≥ 125/min	
• Chronic renal dz.	• Respiratory rate ≥ 30/min	
• Chronic liver dz.	• Systolic blood pressure <90 mmHg	
• Cerebrovas-cular dz.	• Temp < 35°C or > 40°C	
Risk Factor Table		**Points**
Demographic factors		
✔ Age of men		Age (year)
✔ Age of women		Age (year)–10
✔ Nursing home resident		10
Coexisting illnesses		

TABLE 7–26 (Continued)	
✔ Active neoplastic dz.	30
✔ Congestive heart failure	10
✔ Chronic renal dz.	10
✔ Chronic liver dz.	20
✔ Cerebrovascular dz.	10
Physical examination findings	
✔ Altered mental status	20
✔ Pulse ≥ 125/min	10
✔ Respiratory rate ≥ 30/min	20
✔ Systolic blood pressure < 90 mmHg	20
✔ Temp < 35°C or > 40°C	15
Lab findings	
✔ Arterial pH < 7.35	30
✔ BUN ≥ 30 mg/dL (11 mmol/L)	20
✔ Sodium < 130 mmol/L	20
✔ Glucose ≥ 250 mg/dL	10
✔ Hematocrit < 30%	10
✔ PaO_2 < 60 mmHg	10
Radiographic findings	
✔ Pleural effusion10	10

(continued)

TABLE 7–26 (Continued)

Disposition of Patient According to the Pneumonia Scale

Class	Score	Interpretation	
II	<70	Class I and II	Treat as outpatient
III	71–90	Class III	Admit for brief observation
IV	91–130	Class IV and V	Inpatient treatment
V	>130		

Reproduced with permission: Fine MJ, Auble TE, Yealy DM, et al. A prediction rule to identify low risk patients with community acquired pneumonia. *N Engl J Med* 1997;336:243–250.

TABLE 7–27: CAP (Community Acquired Pneumonia) In hospital Therapy

- **CAP with risk factors or comorbid conditions, e.g., COPD, DM, ETOH use (not in ICU)**

- Cover → *S. pneumoniae, H. influenzae, Mycoplasma, Legionella, S. aureus*

- Azithromycin IV + ceftriaxone IV 1st line

- Moxifloxacin IV or levofloxacin IV or gatifloxacin 2nd line

Note: Levofloxacin: adjust for creatinine clearance.

- **Nursing home environment (not in ICU)**

- Cover → Gram (–), *E. coli* and anaerobes

- Azithromycin IV + ceftriaxone IV 1st line

- Moxifloxacin IV or levofloxacin IV or gatifloxacin 2nd line

Note: Levofloxacin: adjust for creatinine clearance.

- **Elderly with chronic alcoholism (not in ICU)**

- Cover → Cover *K. pneumoniae*

- Azithromycin IV + ceftriaxone IV 1st line

- Levofloxacin IV or cefepime IV + azithromycin IV 2nd line

Note: Levofloxacin: adjust for creatinine clearance.

- **Severe CAP in a compromised host (previous admission with MRSA or resides in community with high incidence of MRSA)**

- Vancomycin IV + moxifloxacin IV 1st line

- Moxifloxacin IV + linezolid IV 1st line

- Vancomycin IV + levofloxacin IV 2nd line

(continued)

TABLE 7–27 (Continued)

- **Pneumonia (aspiration)**

- Cover → Gram (–) and anaerobes

- Azithromycin IV + ceftriaxone IV + clindamycin IV 1st line

- Levofloxacin IV + clindamycin IV 2nd line

- Levofloxacin IV + metronidazole 2nd line

- Gatifloxacin IV + clindamycin IV 2nd line

Note: Patient can be discharged on amoxicillin–clavulanate 875 mg PO bid if required.

- **CAP with severe pneumonia requiring ICU admission (*Pseudomonas* is not suspected)**

- Levofloxacin IV + ceftriaxone IV 1st line

- Ceftriaxone IV + moxifloxacin IV 1st line

- Ceftriaxone IV + azithromycin IV 2nd line

- **CAP with severe pneumonia requiring ICU admission (*Pseudomonas* is suspected)**

- Ciprofloxacin IV + ceftazidime IV + azithromycin IV 1st line

- Levofloxacin IV + imipenem IV + aminoglycoside IV 1st line

- Ceftazidime IV + azithromycin IV + aminoglycoside 2nd line

- Moxifloxacin IV + imipenem IV + aminoglycoside IV 2nd line

TABLE 7–27 (Continued)

- **Nosocomial pneumonia (no ICU)**

- Ceftriaxone or cefotaxime or cefuroxime + levofloxacin or moxifloxacin or gatifloxacin or

- Azithromycin or clarithromycin or

- Timentin or ceftriaxone or ceftazidime + gentamicin or tobramycin

    → Covers → Gram (–), *S. aureus*, anaerobes, *S. pneumoniae*, *H. influenzae*

    → If *S. aureus* is prominent in sputum (Gram stain) → add vancomycin IV

Note: IV vancomycin should not be used for >72 h except

1. >1 positive blood Cx β-lactam-resistant coag(–) staph

2. ORSA (oxacillin-resistant *S. aureus*) infection as opposed to colonization

3. β-Lactam-resistant coag (–) infection

4. Serious PCN allergy

- **Nosocomial pneumonia (ICU)**

- Cefepime or

- Ceftazidime or + levofloxacin or moxifloxacin or gatifloxacin

- Ticarcillin/clavulanic acid (Timentin) or

- Piperacillin/tazobactam (Zosyn) azithromycin or clarithromycin

Source with permission: ASCAP (Antibiotic Selection for Community Acquired Pneumonia guideline) 2004. Recommended by other than ASCAP 2004.

TABLE 7–28: Prostatitis

Prostatitis (Acute)

IV agents → Ciprofloxacin 400 mg IV q12h × 2 weeks 1st line

→ Levofloxacin (Levaquin) 500 mg IV daily × 2 weeks 1st line

→ Gatifloxacin 400 mg IV daily × 2 weeks 1st line

→ TMP–SMX 2.5 mg/kg IV q6h × 2 weeks 1st line

→ Aztreonam 2 g IV q8h × 2 weeks 2nd line

PO agents → Ciprofloxacin XR 1000 mg PO daily × 2 weeks 1st line

→ Doxycycline 200 mg PO q12h × 3 days then 100 mg PO daily × 11 days 1st line

→ TMP–SMX SS (single strength) PO daily × 2 weeks 1st line

Prostatitis (chronic)

PO agents → Ciprofloxacin 500 mg PO bid × 1–3 months 1st line

→ Levofloxacin 500 mg PO daily × 1 month 1st line

→ Doxycycline 100 mg PO daily × 1–3 months 1st line

→ TMP–SMX DS (double strength) PO bid × 1–3 months 2nd line

TABLE 7–29: Pyelonephritis

Acute Uncomplicated Pyelonephritis

• Flank pain	• Costovertebral angle tenderness
• Nausea/vomiting	• Presence or absence of cystitis symptoms
• Fever (>38ºC)	• Costovertebral angle tenderness
• Presence or absence of cystitis symptoms	

Lab/Studies

• UA → pyuria, hematuria	• ↑ C-reactive protein
• CBC → leukocytosis	• CT abdomen
• ↑ ESR	• Ultrasound abdomen

Management

• Empiric Rx for Acute Uncomplicated Pyelonephritis

Parenteral	Oral
• Ceftriaxone 1 g IV q24h or	• Ciprofloxacin 500 mg PO bid or
• Ciprofloxacin 200–400 mg IV q12h or	• Ciprofloxacin XR 1000 mg PO daily or
• Levofloxacin 250–500 mg IV q24h or	• Levofloxacin 250–500 mg PO daily or
• Ofloxacin 200–400 mg IV q24h or	• Ofloxacin 200–300 mg PO bid or

(continued)

TABLE 7–29 (Continued)	
• Gatifloxacin 400 mg IV q24h	• Gatifloxacin 400 mg PO daily or
	• Norfloxacin 400 mg PO bid or
	• Lomefloxacin 400 mg PO daily or
	• Enoxacin 400 mg PO bid
• **Empiric Rx for Acute Complicated Pyelonephritis**	
• Cefepime 1 g IV q12h or	
• Ciprofloxacin 400 mg IV q12h or	
• Levofloxacin 500 mg IV q24h or	
• Ofloxacin 400 mg IV q12h or	
• Gatifloxacin 400 mg IV q24h or	
• Gentamicin 3–5 mg/kg IV q24h + ampicillin 1–2 g IV q6h or	
• Gentamicin 1 mg/kg IV q8h + ampicillin 1–2 g IV q6h or	
• Ticarcillin–clavulanate 3.2 g IV q8h or	
• Piperacillin–tazobactam 3.375 g q6-8h or	
• Imipenem–cilastatin 250–500 mg q6-8h	

TABLE 7–29 (Continued)

- **Empiric Rx for Acute Pyelonephritis in Pregnancy**
- Ceftriaxone 1 g IV q24h or
- Gentamicin 1 mg/kg IV q8h + ampicillin 1–2 g IV q6h or
- Ticarcillin–clavulanate 3.2 g IV q8h or
- Aztreonam 1 g IV q8-12h or
- Piperacillin–tazobactam 3.375 g Q6-8h or
- Imipenem–cilastatin 250–500 mg q6-8h

TABLE 7–30: Sexually Transmitted Diseases (STDs)

Gonorrhea	Chlamydia
• Ceftriaxone 125 mg IM × 1 dose 1st line	• Azithromycin 1 g PO × 1 dose 1st line
• Cefixime 400 mg PO × 1 dose or	• Doxycycline 100 mg PO bid × 7 days or
• Ciprofloxacin 500 mg PO × 1 dose or	• Ofloxacin 300 mg PO × 7 days or
• Ofloxacin 400 mg PO × 1 dose or	• Levofloxacin 500 mg daily × 7 days or
• Levofloxacin 250 mg PO × 1 dose or	• Erythromycin 500 mg PO qid × 7 days
• Spectinomycin 40 mg/kg up to 2 g × 1 dose (useful if patient is allergic to ceftriaxone)	

Note: If patient has gonorrhea assume the patient has chlamydia also; thus treat patient for gonorrhea as well as chlamydia. Sexual partners also need to be treated.

Herpes Simplex	Syphilis (Primary/ Secondary/Early Latent)
• Acyclovir 400 mg PO tid × 10 days or	• Benzathine PCN 2.4 million units IM × 1 dose or
• Valacyclovir 1 g PO bid × 10 days or	• Doxycycline 100 mg PO bid × 2 weeks or
• Famciclovir 250 mg PO tid × 10 days	• Erythromycin 500 mg PO qid × 2 weeks

TABLE 7–30 (Continued)	
PID	**Syphilis (Late Latent)**
• Doxycycline 200 mg IV q12h × 3 days then 100 mg IV q12h × 11days + [Cefoxitin 2 g IV q6h × 2weeks or Cefotetan 2 g IV q12h × 2 weeks or Ertapenem 1 g IV daily × 3–10 days]	• Benzathine PCN 2.4 million units IM × 3 weeks or
	• Doxycycline 100 mg PO bid × 4 weeks
	Syphilis (Neurosyphilis)
	• PCN G 3–4 million units IV q4h 10–14 days
• Moxifloxacin 400 mg IV daily × 2 weeks	• Procaine PCN 2.4 million units IM bid × 10–14 days + probenecid 500 mg PO q6h × 10–14 days
• Doxycycline 200 mg IV q12h × 3 days then 100 mg IV q12h × 11 days + Unasyn 3 g IV q6h × 2 weeks	• Ceftriaxone 1 g IV daily × 10–14 days
	• Doxycycline 100 mg PO bid × 10–14 days

TABLE 7–31: Treatment for Pelvic Inflammatory Disease

- Cefotetan 2 g IM q12h or cefoxitin 2 g IV q6h + doxycycline 100 mg IV/PO q12h or

- Clindamycin 900 mg IV q8h + gentamicin or

- Ofloxacin 400 mg IV q12h or levofloxacin 500 mg IV daily ± metronidazole 500 mg IV q8h or

- Ampicillin–Sulbactam 3 g IV q6h + doxycycline 100 mg IV/PO q12h

Source with permission: Center for Disease Control (CDC).

TABLE 7–32: Sinusitis

- Amoxicillin 500 mg PO tid or 875 mg PO bid × 10–14 days 1st line

- Bactrim DS PO bid × 10–14 days 1st line

- Cefpodoxime 200 mg PO bid × 10–14 days 1st line

- Telithromycin (Ketek) 800 mg PO daily × 7–10 days 1st line (if penicillin allergy)

- Cefdinir 600 mg PO daily × 7–10 days 1st line

- Augmentin XR 1 tab bid × 10 days 2nd line

- Levofloxacin (Levaquin) 500–750 mg PO/IV daily × 10 days 2nd line

- Moxifloxacin (Avelox) 400 mg PO/IV daily × 10 days 2nd line

- Gatifloxacin (Tequin) 400 mg PO/IV daily × 10 days 2nd line

TABLE 7–33: Tinea

- **Tinea capitis (scalp ringworm)**

- Griseofulvin (>2 years) 20–25 mg/kg/day divided into bid or daily (take with milk, eggs, or fatty foods)

- Take until 2 weeks after resolution or

- Terbinafine (Lamisil) × 4–6 weeks → if < 20 kg → 67.5 mg/kg PO daily or

- If 20–40 kg → 125 mg PO daily

- If > 40 kg → 250 mg PO daily

- Take until 2 weeks after resolution of the lesion

- Also use selenium sulfide 1–2.5% shampoo in conjunction with medication

- **Tinea corporis (body ringworm)**

- Miconazole 2% topical (cream, lotion, ointment) × 4 weeks or

- Clotrimazole 1% topical cream × 4 weeks or

- Terbinafine (Lamisil) 1% cream apply daily–bid × 2 weeks

- **Tinea versicolor**

- Selenium sulfide shampoo 1–2.5% or

- Terbinafine (Lamisil) 1% solution apply bid until resolved (spray pump solution 1% 30 mL)

(continued)

TABLE 7–33 (Continued)

- **Tinea unguium (nail ringworm)**

- Terbinafine (Lamisil) × 6 weeks → if < 20 kg 67.5 mg/kg PO daily or

- If 20–40 kg 125 mg PO daily

- If > 40 kg 250 mg PO daily

- Itraconazole 3–5 mg/kg/day divided bid or daily × 3 months or

- Fluconazole loading dose 10 mg/kg PO then 3–6 mg/kg/day PO 3–6 months

Note: Treat for 6 weeks for fingernail and 12 weeks for toenail.

TABLE 7–34: Urinary Tract Infection

- **Uncomplicated—treat for 7–10 days**

- TMP–SMX–DS 1 tab PO bid × 3 days 1st line

- Nitrofurantoin 100 mg PO q12h 1st line

- Fosfomycin (Monurol) one 3 g packet PO × 1 dose 1st line

- Augmentin 500 mg PO q12h 1st line

- Ciprofloxacin 250 bid × 3 days or ciprofloxacin 500 daily × 3 days 2nd line

- Levofloxacin 250 mg PO daily × 3 days 2nd line

- Ofloxacin 200 mg PO bid × 3 days 2nd line

- Gentamicin 1 mg/kg IV q8h × 3 days 2nd line

- Ticarcillin–clavulanate 3.2 g IV q8h × 3 days 2nd line

- **Complicated UTI**

- Ampicillin 1 g IV q6h + gentamicin 1 mg/kg IV q8h × 2–3 weeks 1st line

- Zosyn 3.1 g IV q4-6h × 2–3 weeks 2nd line

- Ticarcillin–clavulanate 3.2 g IV q8h × 2–3 weeks 2nd line

- Ceftriaxone 1–2 g IV daily × 2–3 weeks or

- TMP–SMX 800 mg PO bid × 2–3 weeks 1st line

- Norfloxacin 400 mg PO bid × 2–3 weeks 1st line

- Ciprofloxacin 500 mg PO bid × 2–3 weeks 1st line

TABLE 7–35: Vaginitis

Candidiasis (KOH Slide)	Trichomoniasis (NS Slide)	Bacterial (NS Slide)
• White curdy	• Profuse green-gray	• Grey
• pH < 4.5	• pH > 4.5	• pH > 4.5
• Pruritic, burning	• Malodorous	• Whiff test, malodorous
• Budding hyphae	• Trichomonads on WM	• Clue cells on WM
• Tx–fluconazole 150 mg PO × 1 dose	• Metronidazole 2 g × 1 dose (500 mg tab × 4), avoid in 1st trimester	• Metronidazole 375 mg PO bid × 7 days
• Itraconazole 200 mg PO bid × 1 day	• Metronidazole 500 mg PO bid × 7 days, avoid in 1st trimester	• Metronidazole 0.75% vaginal gel qhs × 7 days
• Miconazole vaginal cream 2% × 7 days	• Clotrimazole 100 mg 1 tab qhs × 7–14 days	• Clindamycin 300 mg 1 PO bid × 7 days

Note
• Patient with trichomoniasis infection partner/s should also be treated.
• Avoid metronidazole in 1st trimester.
• Do not use fluconazole (Diflucan) in pregnancy.
Abbreviations: WM, wet mount, NS, normal saline.

TABLE 7–36: VRE (Vancomycin-resistant Enterococci)

- **Blood**

- Cubicin (Daptomycin) → CrCl ≥ 30 → 4 mg/kg/day < 30 → 4 mg/kg every other day or

- Synercid (quinupristin + dalfopristin) 7.5 mg /kg IV q12h or

   (SE: QT elongation with cisapride, terfenadine)

- Linezolid (Zyvox) 600 mg IV/PO bid
  (SE: thrombocytopenia)

- **Urine**

- Nitrofurantoin → If CrCl > 30 then 100 mg PO daily, if < 30 avoid using it or

- Doxycycline 200 mg IV/PO daily

8
Nephrology & Electrolytes

TABLE 8–1: Formulas

- Anion gap (8–16) = $Na^+ - (Cl + HCO_3)$

- Plasma osmolality (285 mOsm/kg H_2O) = $2 \times Na^+ + [(Glu/18) + (BUN/2.8)]$

- Plasma tonicity (effective plasma Osmolality [285 mOsm/kg H_2O]) = $2 \times Na^+ + (Glu/18)$

- Osmolal gap (<10) = measured plasma osmolarity – calculated plasma osmolarity

- CrCl (Cockcroft-Gault)

- CrCl for male (97–137 mL/min) = $(140 - age) \times$ wt (kg)/72 × serum creatinine

- CrCl for female (88–128 mL/min) = 0.85 × CrCl of male

- CrCl (MDRD formula)

- GFR (mL/min/1.732) = $170 \times$ (serum creatinine) – $0.999 \times$ (age) – $0.176 \times$ (BUN) – $0.170 \times$ (Alb) + $0.318 \times$ (0.762 if female) × (1.180 if African-American)

- GFR = $(140 - age) \times$ wt (kg)/85 × serum creatinine

TABLE 8–2: Normal Urine Analysis			
• Color	Straw	• Blood	Absent
• Specific gravity	1.001–1.020	• Eosinophil	Absent
• Appearance	Clear	• Glucose	Absent
• PH	4.5–7.5	• Ketones	Absent
• Leukocyte esterase	Absent	• Myoglobin	Absent
• Nitrite	Absent	• Protein	Absent
Microscopic Examination			
• RBC	0–5 hpf (high power field)	• Bacteria	Absent
• WBC	0–5 hpf	• Cast	0–4 lpf (low power field)
Urine Analysis Abnormalities			
↑ Specific gravity	Dehydration, SIADH, DM, adrenal insufficiency		
↓ Specific gravity	Diabetes insipidus, renal disease, IV hydration (excessive fluid)		
↑ pH (>7.5)	Bacteriuria, vegetarian diet, meds: acetazolamide, $NaHCO_3$		
↓ pH	Acidosis, DM, starvation, diarrhea, meds: methenamine mandelate		
Leukocyte esterase +	Indicates there is an inflammatory reaction occurring in urinary tract		
Nitrite +	Indicates presence of bacteria		

TABLE 8–2 (Continued)	
Blood +	Trauma to urinary tract, renal disease, UTI, rhabdo, anticoagulants, ASA
	If UA is (+) for blood perform microscopy for RBCs
Eosinophils +	Interstitial nephritis, acute tubular necrosis (ATN), UTI
	Hepatorenal syndrome, kidney transplant rejection
Glucose +	DM, renal glucosuria, meds: thiazides, corticosteroids, OCP, ACTH
Ketone +	DKA, AKA, starvation, isopropanol ingestion, vomiting, diarrhea
	Acute febrile illness in children
Myoglobin +	Trauma, hyperthermia, polymyositis/dermatomyositis
	Carbon monoxide poisoning, hypothyroidism, muscle ischemia
	Drugs: narcotics and amphetamines
Protein +	Normal is <150 mg/24 h
	Renal disease (nephrotic syndrome, nephritic syndrome, and so on)
	Preeclampsia in pregnancy
	Multiple myeloma, Waldenström's macroglobulin (+SSA)

(continued)

TABLE 8–2 (Continued)	
Urinary Casts	
Broad casts	Advanced renal failure
Epithelial cell casts	Acute tubular necrosis and acute glomerulonephritis
Fatty casts	Composed of cholesterol esters and cholesterol, seen in lipiduria
Granular casts	Advanced renal failure (represents degenerating cellular casts/ aggregated protein)
Hyaline casts	Normal (seen with small volumes of concentrated urine or with diuretic therapy)
Muddy brown casts	Acute tubular necrosis
Red cell casts	Glomerulonephritis or vasculitis
Waxy casts	Advanced renal failure
White cell casts	Tubulointerstitial disease or acute pyelonephritis

TABLE 8–3: Urine Electrolytes	
Urine Sodium (0–300 meq/L)	**Urine Chloride (0–300 meq/L)**
• Needed in calculating FeNa	• Useful in metabolic alkalosis
• Used in evaluation of oliguria	• Used in evaluation of volume status
1. High in acute tubular necrosis	**Urine Potassium (5–300 meq/L)**
2. Dehydration (volume status) ($\downarrow$)	• Used to determine if the kidney is the source of potassium loss
• Used in evaluation of hyponatremia	
Urine Osmolarity (50–1400 Osmol/kgH$_2$O)	**Urine Creatinine (10–400 mg/dL or 0.4–2.5 g/day)**
• Used in evaluation of hyponatremia	
• Used in evaluation of hyperkalemia	• Useful in calculating creatinine clearance
• Used in evaluation of volume status	• Needed in calculating FeNa
Urine anion gap = [(Na) + (K)] – Cl (negative is considered normal)	
• Indicated in hyperchloremic metabolic gap acidosis	

(continued)

TABLE 8–3 (Continued)		
If Negative and Urine pH < 5.5	**If Positive and Urine pH < 5.5**	
A. Normal or exogenous ammonium chloride	A. 1st degree aldosterone deficiency	
If Negative and Urine pH > 5.5	**If Positive and Urine pH > 5.5**	
A. GI bicarbonate loss	A. Classic RTA	
B. Distal RTA	B. Hyperkalemic RTA	
↑ **Urine Osmolality and Serum Osmolality**		
Addison's dz.	Dehydration	Hypercalcemia
Alcohol abuse	DI	Mannitol
Azotemia	DM	Renal dz.
CHF	Hyperglycemia	
↓ **Urine Osmolality and Serum Osmolality**		
Adrenocortical deficiency	SIADH	
Diuretic use	Over hydration	
Hyponatremia	Water intoxication	
Low salt diet		

TABLE 8–4: Acute Renal Failure

Etiology

Prerenal	Intra Renal
• Dehydration	• Prolonged renal ischemia (ATN)
• Shock	• Medications: NSAIDS, amphotericin B, aminoglycosides
• Low cardiac output	• Medication associated with interstitial nephritis (see below)
Postrenal	• Hypercoagulable state
• BPH	• Emboli
• Prostate disease	• Glomerulonephritis
• Kidney stone	
• Pelvic malignancy	

Physical Examination Findings in Renal Failure

Prerenal	Intra Renal	Postrenal
Weight loss or gain	Weight gain	Enlarged prostate
Poor skin turgor	Mental status change	Weight gain
Orthostatic hypotension	Hypotension/hypertension	Bladder distention
Ascites	Increase JVD	Pelvic mass from bladder distention
Edema		

(continued)

TABLE 8–4 (Continued)			
Signs and Symptoms			
• Malaise, anorexia, nausea (from uremia)			
Prerenal	**Intrarenal**		**Postrenal**
UNa^+ (meq/L)	<20	>30	**Acute**
FeNa	<1	>2	May appear like prerenal failure
U/P Cr	>40	<20	
Uosmol	>500	<35	**Chronic**
BUN/Cr ratio	>10:1	10:1	May appear like renal failure

FeNa = (Una/Pna)/(Ucr/Pcr)

Note: Patient with renal failure → monitor weight, urine output, and I/O electrolytes

ARF (intrarenal failure)

• Causes ↑ in K^+, PO_4, Mg and ↓ in Na^+, HCO_3

• Renal US may help with differential

TABLE 8–4 (Continued)

• ATN 2° to myoglobinuria → urine dipstick→ occult blood	
	→ UA microscopy→ no blood
	→ Order CPK (>10,000 for ARF)
	→ Rx: fluid management/protein restriction/monitor K^+/dialysis
	→ Furosemide 1–9 mg/h (loading dose not required)
	→ Alkalinize urine → acetazolamide

Prerenal failure

Rx → volume challenge/maximize cardiac output

Postrenal failure

Rx → catheter drainage/ureteral stent/nephrostomy

TABLE 8–5: Renal Tubular Acidosis (RTA) Etiologies		
I (Distal)	**II (Proximal)**	**IV (Hypoaldosteronism)**
• Medications (amphotericin)	• Acetazolamide	• ↓ Renin: diabetic nephropathy, NSAIDs, interstitial nephritis
• Hepatitis	• Amyloidosis	
• Nephrocalcinosis	• Fanconi's	• ↓ Aldosterone: ACE, ARB, heparin, 1° adrenal disorder
• Multiple myeloma	• Multiple myeloma	
• Sjögren's syndrome		• ↓ Response to aldosterone
• SLE		Meds: TMP–SMX, K-sparing
		Diuretics, pentamidine,
		Tacrolimus
		Interstitial dz.: amyloid, DM, sickle cell, SLE

TABLE 8–5 (Continued)

Renal Tubular Acidosis (RTA)

Type	I (Distal)	II (Proximal)	IV
Etiology	Defect in H^+ secretion	Defect HCO_3 absorption	Hypoaldost-eronism
Urine pH	>6	<6	<6
Plasma K^+	Low	Low	High
Urine NH_4	Low	Normal	Low
Urine AG	(+)	(±)	(+)
Treatment	HCO_3	Diuretic	Diuretic

anion gap

Plasma osmolarity (280–290) = $2 \times Na^+$ + (Glu/18) + (BUN/2.8)

Osmolal gap (<10) = measured plasma osmolarity by lab calculated plasma osmolarity

TABLE 8–6: Drugs Associated with Interstitial Nephritis

• Allopurinol	• Cimetidine	• NSAIDS	• Protonix
• Captopril	• Ciprofloxacin	• PCN	• Rifampin
• Cephalothin	• Furosemide/ Thiazides	• Phenytoin	• TMP–SMX

TABLE 8–7: Chronic Kidney Disease (CKD) Stages

Stage	GFR (mL/min)	Description
0	120–125	Normal kidney
I	90–119	Kidney damage with Normal or increased GFR
II	60–89	Kidney damage with mildly decreased GFR
III	30–59	Kidney damage with moderately decreased GFR
IV	15–29	Kidney damage with severely decreased GFR
V	≤15	Kidney failure/ESRD

CKD treatment modalities

- Tight control of DM and BP, consider low protein diet and consider starting ACE[a]

- Avoid medications that may cause kidney damage

- Electrolyte balance

- Treat anemia

- Dialysis

- Kidney transplant

[a]Do not start ACE if creatinine >3.

TABLE 8–8: Plasma BUN (8–18 mg/dL) and Creatinine(0. 5–1.5 mg/dL)		
↑ **BUN**	↓ **BUN**	↑ **Creatinine**
• Renal failure	• Calorie/protein deficiency	• ARF
• Postrenal obstruction	• ETOH abuse	• CRF
• Dehydration	• Liver dz.	• DKA [false (+)]
• Steroids	• Celiac dz.	• Drugs
• GI bleed	• Acromegaly	Trimethoprim
• High protein diet	• Overhydration	Probenecid
• TPN	• Plasma volume	Cimetidine
• Drugs	1. Pregnancy (3rd trimester)	↓ **Creatinine**
• Amino-glycoside	2. SIADH	• ↓ Muscle mass
• Corticosteroids		
• Diuretics		
• Tetracyclines		

(continued)

TABLE 8–8 (Continued)	
Maintenance Fluid	
1st 10 kg of total body weight	100 mL/kg/day or 4 mL/kg/h
2nd 10 kg of total body weight	50 mL/kg/day or 2 mL/kg/h
Above 20 kg of total body weight	20 mL/kg/day or 1 mL/kg/h
Urinary Output	

- Urine output $\rightarrow$ Adult $\rightarrow$ male = 20–25 mL/kg/24 h
  $\rightarrow$ Female = 15–20 mL/kg/24 h

- Urine output $\rightarrow$ Adult $\rightarrow$ $^1/_2$ mL/kg/h
  $\rightarrow$ Peds $\rightarrow$ 1 mL/kg/h

- Oliguria (UO <400 mL/24 h or 0.5 mL/kg/h)

TABLE 8–9: Electrolyte Corrections

Correction of Na$^+$

- Corrected Na$^+$ for glucose = Na$^+$ + [(Glu − 100) × 0.016]

- Corrected Na$^+$ for glucose = Na$^+$ + [(Glu − 200)/42]

- For each 100 ↑ glucose above 200 mg/dL → Na$^+$ ↓ by 1.6

- Corrected Na$^+$ for triglyceride (meq/L) = plasma TG (g/L) × 0.002

- Corrected Na$^+$ for albumin (meq/L) = (albumin [g/L]−8) × 0.025

Correction of K$^+$

- For change in pH of 0.1 → K$^+$ changes inversely 0.5 − 1.2 meq/L

Correction of Ca

- Corrected Ca for albumin = [0.8 × (4 − patient's albumin) + Ca]

- For q1g/dL of albumin, Ca by 0.8 mg/dL

Correction of HCO$_3$

- Corrected HCO$_3$ for anion gap = HCO$_3$ + (anion gap − 12)

Correction of anion gap

- ↓ Albumin 1 g = ↓ anion gap by ≈ 2.2–2.5

TABLE 8–10: Total Body Water and Sodium Distribution in Hypo- and Hypernatremia

ECF Volume	Total Body Na$^+$	TBW(Free)	
• Hyponatremia			
↓	↓↓	↓	Hypovolemic
N	N	↑	Isovolemic
↑	↑	↑↑	Hypervolemic
• Hypernatremia			
↓	↓	↓↓	Hypovolemic
N	N	↓	Isovolemic
↑	↑↑	↑	Hypervolemic
Abbreviation: N, normal			

TABLE 8–11: Hyponatremia (<135 meq/L)

Etiology

• Diuretic therapy	• Cerebral salt wasting
• Nephropathy/ATN/nephrotic syndrome	• Third spacing (burn, ascites)
• Adrenal insufficiency	• Glucocorticoid deficiency
• Metabolic alkalosis	• Hypothyroidism
• Pseudohypoaldosteronism	• CHF

Pseudohyponatremia

• 2° to $\uparrow$ plasma glucose, hypothyroidism, high lipid and high protein

Correction of sodium

• Corrected Na^+ for glucose = $Na^+ + [(Glu - 100) \times 0.016]$

• Corrected Na^+ for glucose = $Na^+ + [(Glu - 200)/42]$

• For each $100 \uparrow$ glucose above 200 mg/dL $\rightarrow Na^+ \downarrow$ by 1.6

• Corrected Na^+ for triglyceride (meq/L) = plasma TG (g/L) $\times$ 0.002

• Corrected Na^+ for albumin (meq /L) = [albumin (g/L) – 8] $\times$ 0.025

Hyponatremia investigation

• **Isovolemic** $\rightarrow$ Differential $\rightarrow$ SIADH, hypothyroidism, cortisol deficiency, thiazide

• Check urine Na^+ level (meq/L)

(continued)

TABLE 8–11 (Continued)

- Urine Na$^+$ < 10 meq/L → water intoxication

- Urine Na$^+$ > 20 meq/L → SIADH, diuretic induced

- Rx → water restriction to 500–1000 mL/day

- **Hypovolemic** (patient appears dry) → check urine Na$^+$ level (meq/L)

- If urine Na$^+$ > 20 meq/L → 2° to diuresis, mineralocorticoid defficiency, RTA

- If urine Na$^+$ < 20 meq/L → diarrhea, vomiting, third spacing

- Rx → symptomatic → 3% saline

- Asymptomatic patient → 0.9% saline (200–250 mL/h of 1 L then 125–150 mL/h)

- **Hypervolemic** (edema) → check urine Na$^+$ level (meq/L)

- If urine Na$^+$ < 20 meq/L → heart failure, cirrhosis, nephrosis

- If urine Na$^+$ > 20 meq/L → renal failure

- Rx → water restriction to 500–1000 mL/day

Note: Also see Table 8–3.

Calculating Sodium Deficit in Hypovolemic Hyponatremia

- Na$^+$ concentration in IV fluids → 3% saline = 513 meq/L, NS 154 meq/L, $\frac{1}{2}$ NS 75 meq/L

1. TBW (L) = 0.5 × wt (kg)

2. Na$^+$ concentration deficit (meq/L) = 130 – current Na$^+$ level (meq/L)

TABLE 8–11 (Continued)

3. Na^+ deficit (meq) = TBW × (Na^+ concentration deficit)

4. Fluid to be infused → 3% saline → has 513 meq/L of Na^+, NS 154 meq Na^+

5. Volume to be infused (mL) = (Na^+ deficit/Na^+ meq/L in solution) × 1000

6. Total hours for correction of sodium deficit = Na^+ concentration deficit/0.5 ← (the speed of correction of Na^+ [meq/L/h])

7. Rate of infusion = volume to be infused/hours for the infusion

Note: Do not correct the rise in plasma Na^+ > 0.5 meq/L/h or 12 meq/24 h. Correct to 130 meq/L.

Example

1. A 60 kg female with Na^+ level of = 120 meq/L

2. TBW (L) = (0.5 × 60) → 30 L

3. Na^+ concentration deficit = 130 − 120 → 10 meq/L

4. Na^+ deficit (meq) = (30 L) × (10 meq/L) → 300 meq

5. Fluid to be infused → 3% saline → 513 meq/L of Na^+

6. Volume to be infused (mL) = (300/513) × 1000 → 585 mL

Note → Do not correct the rise in plasma Na^+ to 0.5 meq/L/h or up to 130 meq/L.

7. Total hours for correction of sodium deficit = [(10 meq/L)/(0.5 meq/L)] → 20 h

8. Rate of infusion = 585 mL/20 h → 29 mL/h

(continued)

TABLE 8–11 (Continued)
Note
• When correcting hyponatremia the rate of rise in plasma Na^+ should not exceed 0.5 meq/L/h or exceed 12 meq/L/24 h. Do not exceed plasma Na^+ 130 meq/L.
• A major complication is central pontine myelinolysis (aka osmotic demyelination) → which occurs due to rapid correction of sodium, this can be accompanied by pituitary damage and cause oculomotor nerve palsy.
• Si/Sx of central pontine myelinolysis are diplopia, confusion, delirium, dysphagia, dysarthria, muscle spasm, paralysis, weakness, and coma.

TABLE 8–12: Hypernatremia (>145 meq/L)	
Etiology	
• Dehydration	• Hyperaldosteronism
• Diarrhea	• Cushing's syndrome
• Obstructive uropathy	• Diabetes insipidus
• Renal dysplasia	• Excess sodium bicarbonate
• Diabetes mellitus	

Hypovolemic hypernatremia

- Correct TBW deficit in 48–72 h

- $2°$ to fluid loss $\rightarrow$ Rx $\rightarrow$ replace deficit with D_5W (see replacement of total body water)

- Can give 5% albumin to rapidly restore intravascular volume

Normovolemic hypernatremia

- Most likely $2°$ to DI

- Uosm < 200 $\rightarrow$ central DI $\rightarrow$ vasopressin challenge 5 mg IV $\rightarrow$ should Uosm by 50%

- Uosm = 200–500 $\rightarrow$ nephrogenic diabetes insipidus

- Rx: replace TBW in 48–72 h

Hypervolemic hypernatremia

- $2°$ to $\rightarrow$ hypertonic saline solution/HCO_3 infusion/excessive salt ingestion

- Rx $\rightarrow$ furosemide

Note: Also see Table 8–3.

(continued)

TABLE 8–12 (Continued)
Correction of Hypovolemic Hypernatremia
• Na^+ concentration in IV fluids $\rightarrow$ NS = 154 meq/L, $^1/_2$ NS = 75 meq/L
1. TBW in hypernatremia = (M) = $0.5 \times$ wt (kg), (F) = $0.4 \times$ wt (kg)
2. Current TBW = TBW $\times$ (140/Pna)
3. TBW deficit = TBW – current TBW
4. X = replacement fluid Na^+ (meq)/154
5. Replacement volume (L) = TBW deficit $\times$ [1/(1 – X)]
Example
1. A 70 kg male with plasma sodium of 160 meq/L
2. TBW = $(0.5 \times 70 \text{ kg}) \rightarrow$ 35 L
3. Current TBW = $[35 \times (140/160)] \rightarrow$ 30.6 L
4. TBW deficit = $(35–30.6) \rightarrow$ 4.4 L
5. Replacement fluid $\rightarrow$ X = 75 (meq/L)/154 $\rightarrow$ 0.49
6. Replacement volume (L) = 4.4 (L) $\times$ (1/1–0.49) $\rightarrow$ 8.6 L (replace this deficit in 48–72 h)
Note
• Replacement: Give $^1/_2$ in first 24 h and next half in next 48 h.
• Isotonic fluid (NS) should be used initially when correcting TBW deficit and should be corrected slowly over 48–72 h.
• The serum sodium should not fall > 0.5 meq/L/h (12 meq/day).
• Na^+ concentration in IV fluids $\rightarrow$ NS = 154 meq/L, $^1/_2$ NS = 75 meq/L.

TABLE 8–13: Hypokalemia: Common Etiology	
• Diarrhea/vomiting/laxative induced	• Magnesium depletion
• Pyloric obstruction	• Insulin
• Alkalosis	• RTA I and II
• High renin state	• Cushing's syndrome/disease
• Hyperaldosteronism	• Adrenal hyperplasia (11- and 17-hydroxylase deficiency)
• Chewing tobacco	• Licorice
• Carbenicillin	• Amphotericin B
• Mineralocorticoid (Florinef)	• Diuretic (furosemide, ethacrynic acid)
Correction of K$^+$	
• For change in pH of 0.1 → K$^+$ changes inversely 0.5–1.2 meq/L	
Hypokalemia (<3.5 meq)	
• Check Mg level (if low, correct Mg level prior to correcting K$^+$ level)	
• Mg depletion impairs K$^+$ reabsorption across the renal tubule	

(continued)

TABLE 8–13 (Continued)
A. K-Dur 20–40 meq tab PO bid–qid
B. Micro-K⁺ 10 meq tab PO bid–tid (max 100 meq/day)
C. KCl elixir 1–3 tbs (20 meq in 1 tbs)
D. KCl 10–80 meq in 1 L NS infuse over 2 h
E. KCl 20–40 meq in 100 mL NS infuse over 2 h
• 10 meq KCl in 100 mL NS → can be given via peripheral line over 1 h
• 20 meq KCl in 100 mL NS → can be given via central line over 1 h
Note: 40–60 meq can K⁺ by 1–1.5 meq/L but this may be transient.
Do not give > 10 meq IV qh via peripheral line or >20 meq IV qh via central line.

TABLE 8–14: Hyperkalemia: Common Etiology		
• Metabolic or respiratory acidosis	**Medications**	
• Adrenal insufficiency	• ACE	• K^+ sparing diuretics
• Patient on chronic steroid and the sudden discontinue	• Arginine	• K^+ Penicillin
• Hemolyzed blood	• β-Blocker	• NSAIDs
• Renal failure	• Cyclosporine	• Pentamidine
• Aldosterone antagonist	• Digitalis toxicity	• Succinylcholine
• Hypoaldosteronism	• Heparin	• THAM
• Blood transfusion	• Insulin	• TMP–SMX
• Thrombocytosis/ leukocytosis		
• Muscle necrosis		
Hyperkalemia (>5 meq/L)		
• $2°$ → Transcellular shift → acidosis/myonecrosis		
→ Blood transfusion (1 unit of whole blood can ↑ K^+ by 0.25 meq/24 h)		
→ √Meds → ACE/heparin/NSAIDs/digitalis/β-blockers/ TMP–SMX/K^+ sparing diuretics		

(continued)

TABLE 8–14 (Continued)
• Recheck K^+ level and check ECG) → if $K^+ > 7$ meq/L or ECG changes
• Check urine K^+ level → if > 30 meq/L → suggests transcellular shift
→ If < 30 meq/L → suggests impaired renal secretion
• Rx → Calcium gluconate: 10 mL of 10% (1 amp) infuse slowly over 2–3 min (onset 2–3 min)
→ Repeat dose in 5 min if ECG changes persists
→ Insulin (regular) 10 units + 50 mL of a 50% glucose solution IV (onset 15–20 min)
→ Albuterol 10–20 mg in 4 mL saline by nasal inhalation over 10 min (onset 30 min)
→ Kayexalate (Na^+ polystyrene) 20 g with 100 mL of 20% sorbitol PO q4-6h
→ To give Kayexalate as enema: 50 g in 50 mL of 70% sorbitol + 150 mL tap H_2O
→ Bicarbonate 45 meq (1 amp of 7.5% $NaHCO_3$) IV over 5 min (onset 30 min)
→ Epinephrine 0.05 µg/kg/min IV (onset 30 min)
→ If no response to above Rx or severe hyperkalemia → consider dialysis
Note: Kayexalate is contraindicated in bowel obstruction.

TABLE 8–14 (Continued)

TTKG (transtubular potassium gradient): normal 8–9 (can be up to 12 in K^+ rich diet)

- $TTKG = (U_{K^+} \times P_{osm})/(P_{K^+} \times U_{osm})$

- In patient with hypokalemia, without any disease TTKG should be < 3

- In patient with hypokalemia, without any disease and TTKG > 3 → renal loss of K^+

- In patient with hyperkalemia, without any disease TTKG should be > 10

- Patient with hyperkalemia and TTKG of < 7 → indicates hypoaldosteronism/renal tubular defect

Note: Hypoaldosteronism: Administration of mineralocorticoid 9 α-fludrocortisone 0.05 mg should cause → TTKG to rise > 7.

Causes of Hyperkalemia (Not Responding to Mineralocorticoid Challenge)

• K^+ sparing diuretics	• Tubular resistance to aldosterone
Amiloride	Interstitial Nephritis
Spironolactone	Sickle disease
Triamterene	Urinary tract obstruction
• Drugs	Pseudohypoaldosteronism type I
Trimethoprim	• ↑ distal nephron K^+ reabsorption
Pentamidine	• Pseudohypoaldosteronism type I

TABLE 8–15: Hypomagnesemia (<1.3 meq/L): Etiology

Urinary Loss	Intestinal Loss	Miscellaneous
Hypercalcemia	Malabsorption	Alcoholism
Hyperglycemia	Laxative use	Sepsis
Hypophosphatemia	Pancreatitis	Malnutrition
RTA (renal tubular acidosis)	Severe diarrhea	Metabolic acidosis
	Intestinal and biliary fistula	Acute MI
Meds		Thermal injury
Aminoglycosides	Cyclosporine	Hyperthyroidism
Amphotericin-B	Digitalis	Diabetes
β Agonist	Diuretics	Hypoalbumin
Cisplatin	Insulin	TPN
Catecholamine	Pentamidine	Citrated blood product

- Mg deficit = $0.2 \times$ wt (kg) $\times$ desired $\uparrow$ in Mg concentration $\rightarrow$ replace within 2–3 days

Note: Monitor respiratory drive and tendon reflexes when replacing Mg.

TABLE 8–15 (Continued)

• Rx → MgO × 400 or 600 mg PO (600 mg provides 35 meq) 1–2 tablets daily
→ MgCl 65–130 mg PO tid–qid (64 mg = 5.3 meq/tab)
→ Severe (<1 mg/dL) → MgSO$_4$ 1–6 g in 500 mL D$_5$W at 1 g/h
Note: Sulfate can cause metabolic acidosis if used for a long period of time.

Symptoms and Signs	
• Arrhythmia	• Angina
• Weakness	• Tremors
• Confusion	• Nausea

TABLE 8–16: Hypermagnesemia (>2.4 meq/L)

• Check ECG (↑ PR, ↑ QRS)
• Rx → Saline diuresis → NS or ½ NS at 100–300 mL/h
→ CaCl 1–3 g in IVF at 1 g/h
→ Furosemide 20–40 mg IV q4-6h
→ (If Mg > 9) → stat hemodialysis

TABLE 8–17: Hypocalcemia and Hypercalcemia

- Calcium (8.8–10.3 mg/dL; 4.4–5.2 meq/L; 2.2–2.6 mmol/L)

- ↓ Albumin 1 g = ↓ Ca 0.8 mg/dL (0.2 mmol/L)

- Corrected [Ca] = Measured total [Ca] mg/dL + [0.8 × (4.5 − [albumin] g/dL)]

Hypocalcemia: Etiology

• Hypoalbuminemia	• Hyperphosphatemia
• Hypomagnesemia	• Recent use of MRI with Gadolinium
• Excess fluoride	• Vitamin D deficiency
• Pancreatitis	• Renal insufficiency
• Alkalosis	• Sepsis

Note: Large volume of blood transfusion → citrate used as an anticoagulant chelates calcium

• Drugs	Foscarnet	Ethylene diamine tetracetate (EDTA)	Citrate
	Heparin	Cimetidine	Aminoglycosides
	Cisplatin	Leucovorin	Corticosteroid

TABLE 8–17 (Continued)	
Hypocalcemia Symptoms	
• Paresthesia	• Tetany
• Hypotension	• Seizure
• Chvostek's sign	• Trousseau's sign
• Bradycardia	• Prolongation of QT interval

Acute Hypocalcemia Treatment

- Calcium chloride (CaCl) 10% (270 mg calcium/10 mL vial) give 5–10 mL over 10 min

- CaCl 10% (270 mg calcium/10 mL vial) dilute in 50–100 mL D_5W over 20–30 min

- Calcium gluconate 20 mL of 10% (2 vials) infused over 10–15 min followed by infusion of 60 mL in 500 mL of D_5W at 0.5–2 mg/kg/h

Chronic Hypocalcemia Treatment

- Calcium carbonate (Oscal) 1–2 tab PO tid, calcium citrate (Citracal) 1 tab PO q8h

- Vitamin D_2 (Ergocalciferol) 1 tab PO daily

- Calcitriol 0.25 μg PO daily titrate up to 0.5–2 μg qid

- Docusate sodium (Colace) 1 tab PO bid

(continued)

TABLE 8–17 (Continued)	
Hypercalcemia Management	
To ↑ Excretion	**To ↓ Intestinal Absorption**
• Loop diuretic + NS	• Phosphate PO in chronic hypercalcemia
• Furosemide 20–80 mg IV q4-12h + NS 1–2 L/1–4 h then 125—150 mL/h	• Corticosteroid in hypervitaminosis D
To ↓ Bone Resorption	**To ↑ Chelate Ionized Calcium**
• Calcitonin (Calcimar)	• EDTA
• Gallium nitrate	• Phosphate IV
• Bisphosphonates (Aredia 30–90 g/day)	• Phosphate PO
Note: Dialysis if all Rx fails.	

TABLE 8–18: Hypophosphatemia: Symptoms and Signs

• Weakness	• Respiratory muscle paralysis
• Confusion	• Neurological dysfunction
• Myopathy	• RBC hemolysis

Hypophosphatemia (<2.5 mg/dL) Management

• If (>1) → Neutra-Phos capsule 250 mg 2 tab PO bid or tid
→ Phospho-Soda 5 mL PO bid or tid (5 mL = 129 mg phosphorus)
• If (<1) → 0.08–0.16 mmol/kg over 6 h until phosphorus level is 1.5 mg/dL
→ Na-Phosphate or K^+-Phosphate 10 mmol in 250 mL NS or D_5W over 8 h
Note: Rapid replacement with phosphorus can cause hypocalcemia (monitor for signs: tetany)
If K^+ level is < 3.5 use K^+-Phosphate, otherwise use Na-Phosphate

TABLE 8–19: Hyperphosphatemia (>4.5 mg/dL) Management

- **Mild–moderate**

  - Ca–carbonate 1 g with each meal

  - Insulin and glucose (cell phosphate uptake) is used when rapid ↓ in phosphate is needed

  - Al-Hydroxide (Amphojel) 5–10 mL or 1–2 tab PO ac (before meals) tid

  - Al-Carbonate (Basalgel) 5–10 mL or 1–2 tab PO ac (before meals) tid

- **Severe → NS 1–3 L over 1–3 h**

  → Acetazolamide (Diamox) 500 mg PO or IV q6h

  → Dialysis

9
Neurology

TABLE 9–1: Neurology Terminology

- Abulia: apathy, lack of impulse to action, expressionless face (due to frontal lobe defect)

- Acalculia: inability to calculate

- Agnosia: impairment of recognition of objects, people, shapes, sounds, and smells

  - Anosognosia: unaware of neurological deficit (due to parietotemporal lesion)

  - Object agnosia: impairment of recognition of objects

  - Neglect: disregards stimuli from one side of the body

- Agraphia: inability to express thought in written language

- Alexia: inability to understand written language

- Aphasia: difficulty with language production (inability to use or understand words)

  - Lesion is in the dominant hemisphere

  - Broca's aphasia (productive): nonfluent speech, intact comprehension, impaired repetition (lesion in inferior frontal gyrus)

  - Wernicke's (receptive): impaired comprehension, fluent speech with paraphasic errors, and impaired repetition (lesion in superior temporal gyrus)

  - Conductive aphasia: relatively normal speech, striking deficit of repetition (lesion in superior temporal or inferior parietal region)

(continued)

TABLE 9–1 (Continued)
• Apraxia: inability to perform task due to cognition and not due to motor dysfunction
• Ideomotor apraxia: disordered sequence of complex movement (unable to perform simple tasks)
• Constructional apraxia: disorder of spatial design or drawing (difficulty in manipulating objects in space)
• Dysarthria: disorder of articulation of sounds
• Echopraxia: imitating actions
• Echolalia: repeating words
• Palilalia: involuntary repetition of phrase with increasing velocity (Parkinson's disease).

TABLE 9–2: Cranial Nerves

Olfactory nerve

   A. Test smell with coffee, soap, or alcohol swab

Optic nerve

   A. Test visual acuity/visual fields

   B. Test peripheral vision

   C. Ophthalmologic examination

Oculomotor nerve

   A. Test all EOM

(All are innervated by CN III except lateral rectus and superior oblique (SO4 LR6)

Superior oblique by CN 4 and lateral rectus by CN 6

   B. Test direct and consensual pupillary reflex

Trochlear nerve

   A. Test superior oblique (function: downward and inward movement of the eye)

Trigeminal nerve

   A. Test facial sensory: (1) V_1 ophthalmic, (2) V_2 maxillary, and (3) V_3 mandibular

   B. Test corneal reflex

   C. Test muscles of mastications (bite, jaw opening)

Abducens nerve

   A. Test lateral rectus (function: lateral deviation of the eye)

(continued)

TABLE 9–2 (Continued)

Facial nerve

A. Test facial muscles of expression: smile, frown, raise, and close eyebrows
B. Test taste anterior $2/3$ of tongue

Vestibulocochlear nerve

A. Test hearing with rubbing fingers around the ear or with tuning fork
B. Test balance

Glossopharyngeal nerve and vagus nerve

A. Test gag reflex (touch soft palate or pharynx)
B. Test swallowing
C. Check for position of uvula
D. Test posterior $1/3$ of tongue

Accessory nerve

A. Test trapezius muscle strength (have patient shrug shoulder)
B. Test sternocleidomastoid muscle strength (lateral head rotation against resist)

Hypoglossal nerve

A. Test muscles of tongue

FIGURE 9–1: Extra ocular muscle movement

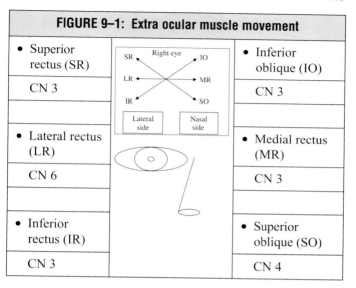

• Superior rectus (SR) CN 3	• Inferior oblique (IO) CN 3
• Lateral rectus (LR) CN 6	• Medial rectus (MR) CN 3
• Inferior rectus (IR) CN 3	• Superior oblique (SO) CN 4

FIGURE 9–2: Dermatomal Map

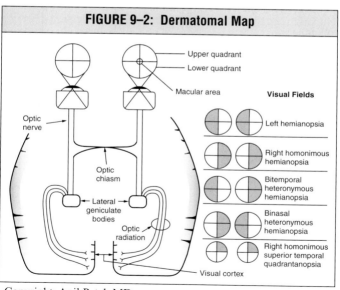

TABLE 9–3: Localization of Pathology in the Brain

Area of the Brain	Pathology
Frontal lobes	Apathy, inattention, labile affect
Dominant frontal lobe	Broca's aphasia (motor)
Temporal lobe	Memory impairment/aggressive sexual behavior
Dominant temporal lobe	Wernicke's aphasia (sensory)
Non-dominant parietal lobe	Difficulty dressing/ignores one side of body
Dominant parietal lobe	Inability to read, write, or perform math
Occipital lobe	Visual hallucination/illusions
Cerebellum	Ataxia, dysarthria, dysmetria, intention tremor, nystagmus, scanning speech
Midbrain	Cranial nerves 3 and 4
Pons	Cranial nerves 5–8
Medulla	Cranial nerves 9–12
Lower motor neuron defect (nerve/muscle)	Decrease or absence of reflex, fasciculations
Upper motor neuron defect (cord/brain)	Hyperreflexia

TABLE 9–4: Lobes and their Functions

Frontal Lobe	Temporal Lobe
Judgment	Emotional response
Organization skills	Memory
Executive function	Location of Wernicke's area
Motivation	
Location of Broca's area	
Parietal Lobe	**Dominant Parietal Lobe**
Perception and interpretation of sensory information	Right to left orientation
Ability to identify object by tactile stimuli	Naming fingers
Visual–spatial sensory (drawing clock, smiley face, or copy pentagon)	Calculation
	Perform skilled motor tasks without any verbal stimuli
Occipital Lobe	
Visual identification	Recognition of shape, color, and objects
Visual fields	

TABLE 9–5: Muscle Examination

- Check for tone

- Check for atrophy

- Check for range of motion

- Grade for strength (see below)

Grading muscle strength

- 0/5 → No muscle contraction noted

- 1/5 → Muscle contraction, visible or palpable but no movement

- 2/5 → Movement with gravity eliminated

- 3/5 → Movement against gravity only

- 4/5 → Movement against gravity with some resistance

- 5/5 → Movement against gravity with full resistance (normal muscle strength)

Grading deep tendon reflexes

- 0 → Absent reflex

- 1+ → Hypoactive

- 2+ → Normal

- 3+ → Brisker than average

- 4+ → Hyperactive

TABLE 9–5 (Continued)

Coordination—cerebellar function

- Finger to nose
- Rapid alternation movements of hands
  - Finger tapping (index finger to thumb)
  - Wrist rotation
  - Front–back patting (supination and pronation)
- Heel to shin
- Rapid alternating movement of foot
  - Tap foot on examiners palm and then on the floor
- Rapid alternating movement of tongue, lip, and palate
  - Ask patient to repeat lah-lah-lah, pah-pah-pah, and kah-kah-kah
- Check for tremors (ask patient to outstretch their hands parallel to ground)
- Gait → static (normal standing)
  - → Natural ambulation
  - → Tandem gait
  - → Walking on heels and toes
  - → Type of gaits (see below)

	Ataxic	Diplegic	Myopathic
	Choreiform	Neuropathic	Parkinsonism

(continued)

TABLE 9–5 (Continued)

- Romberg sign

  - Have patient stand with arms aligned to side of the hips with eyes open and then close for 20–30 s (stand close enough to support patient to prevent a fall

  - If patient. sways with eyes closed but not with eyes open → it is Romberg (+)

  - A positive test → problem with proprioception and vestibular

TABLE 9–6: Posterior Column Lesion

1. Proprioception

- Have patient close his eyes and move his big toe toward dorsi flex and plantar flex and ask the patient to state whether the toe is up or down

- If patient is inconsistent with answers → proprioceptive problem

- Conditions that commonly causes proprioceptive problems

  A. Multiple sclerosis

  B. Pernicious anemia

  C. Neurosyphilis

2. Stereognosis

- Have the patient close both his eyes

- Place an object on patient's hand like a key, pen, watch, or a coin

- Patient should be able to recognize most of the objects

3. Number-writing (follow the three-step command below)

  A. Take patient's palm

  B. With a blunt object draw a number like "5"

  C. Patient should be able to recognize number writing

(continued)

TABLE 9–6 (Continued)		
Glasgow Coma Scale		
Eye Opening	**Verbal Response**	**Motor Response**
1 = No response	1 = No response	1 = No response to pain
2 = Opens with pain	2 = Unintelligible sounds	2 = Extension with pain (decerebrate)
3 = Opens with verbal stimuli	3 = Inappropriate responses	3 = Flexion with pain (decorticate)
4 = Opens spon-taneously	4 = Converse but confused	4 = Withdraws from pain stimuli
	5 = Alert and oriented	5 = Localization of pain (pushes away)
		6 = Responds to verbal commands
Brainstem reflexes (to determine brainstem function)		
• Corneal reflex		
• Pupillary reflex		
• Gag reflex		
• Doll's eye		
• Cold caloric test (oculovestibular reflex)		

TABLE 9–7: Motor Pathway Defect (Corticospinal Tract)

Upper Motor Neuron Defect	Lower Motor Neuron Defect
• Pathway above synapse in spinal cord	• Pathway after synapse in spinal cord
• Muscle tone increased or spastic	• Muscle tone decreased or flaccid
• Hyperreflexia	• Hyporeflexia
• No fasciculation	• Fasciculation
• No fibrillation	• Fibrillation
• No considerable muscle atrophy	• Considerable muscle atrophy
• May have Babinski reflex (extension of toe)	• Babinski not present (flexion of toe)
• Sustained clonus	• Clonus not present
Note: Metabolic encephalopathy can cause asterixis and myoclonus.	

TABLE 9–8: Other Reflexes

- Babinski reflex: positive if stroking ventral surface of the feet can cause the first (big) toe to extend

- Glabellar reflex: tapping over the forehead responds in closing both eyes

- Palmomental reflex: stroking the palm of the hand causes the ipsilateral mentalis muscle to contract

  (Palmomental reflex and root reflex are inhibited by functioning frontal lobe)

- Root reflex: gently stroking lateral aspect of upper lip causes the mouth to move toward stimuli

TABLE 9–9: Nerve Root Examination

Nerve Root	Reflex	Motor	Sensory
C6	Bicep	Bicep and wrist extension	Medial arm and hand
C7	Tricep	Tricep and wrist flexion	Middle finger
C8	Finger	Finger flexion	Lateral hand
L4	Knee	Quadriceps	Medial calf
L5		Foot dorsiflexion	Medial foot
S1	Ankle	Foot plantar flexion	Lateral foot

FIGURE 9–3: Dermatomal Map

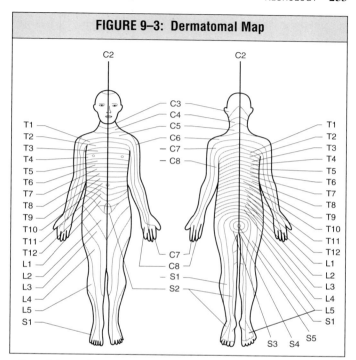

Copyright: Anil Patel, MD

TABLE 9–10: Brain Arterial Supply

Area	Arterial Supply
• Medial cerebral hemisphere (cortex)	Anterior cerebral artery (ACA)
• Lateral cerebral hemisphere (cortex)	Middle cerebral artery (MCA)
• Occipital lobe	Posterior cerebral artery (PCA)
• Superior cerebellum	Superior cerebellar artery (SCA)
• Inferior cerebellum	Anterior inferior cerebellar artery (AICA)
	Posterior inferior cerebellar artery (PICA)
• Pons	Basilar artery (BA)
	Anterior inferior cerebellar artery (ACA)
• Corpus callosum	Anterior cerebral artery (ACA)
• Thalamus	Posterior cerebral artery (PCA)

FIGURE 9–4: Arteries of the Brain

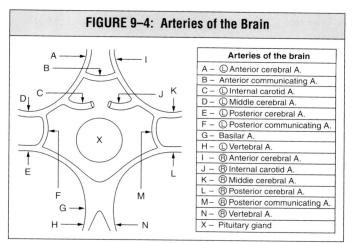

Arteries of the brain
A – Ⓛ Anterior cerebral A.
B – Anterior communicating A.
C – Ⓛ Internal carotid A.
D – Ⓛ Middle cerebral A.
E – Ⓛ Posterior cerebral A.
F – Ⓛ Posterior communicating A.
G – Basilar A.
H – Ⓛ Vertebral A.
I – Ⓡ Anterior cerebral A.
J – Ⓡ Internal carotid A.
K – Ⓡ Middie cerebral A.
L – Ⓡ Posterior cerebral A.
M– Ⓡ Posterior communicating A.
N – Ⓡ Vertebral A.
X – Pituitary giand

TABLE 9–11: Nutrition Deficiencies and Heavy Metal Exposure

Nutrition Deficiencies	Signs and Symptoms
Thiamine (B_1)	Neuropathy, encephalopathy, optic neuropathy
Pyridoxine (B_6)	Neuropathy, seizure
B_{12} and folate	Neuropathy, myelopathy, encephalopathy, optic neuropathy
Vitamin D	Myopathy
Vitamin E	Neuropathy myopathy, myelopathy
Nicotinic acid	Encephalopathy
Heavy Metal Exposure	**Signs and Symptoms**
Arsenic (insecticides)	Sensory and motor neuropathy, red hands, "burning" feet, hyperhydrosis
Lead (paint, gas, batteries)	Adult: neuropathy, arthralgia. Children: cerebral edema, encephalopathy, ↑ IQ
Mercury (polluted fish)	Arm and leg pain, motor neuropathy, dementia
Thallium (insecticides)	Stocking glove sensory motor neuropathy and alopecia

Tube Number	Test for
1	Cell count
2	Gram stain, bacteria, viral, and fungus C&S, AFB, India Ink
3	Glucose, protein, LDH, VDRL
4	Cell count, RBC, WBC
5	Hold for other tests

TABLE 9–12: Lumbar Puncture and Tube Contents

TABLE 9–13: CSF Analysis

	Normal Value		Normal Value
Appearance	Clear/colorless	Cell count	0–5 cells/mm^3
Pressure	70–180 mmH$_2$O	WBC	<5 per mL (<20 in newborn)
Glucose	40–70 mg/dL	Lymphocyte	60–70% (<10)
Protein	<40 mg/dL	Neutrophil	30–50%
Gamma globulin	3–12% of total proteins	Monocyte	None

CSF Analysis and Associated Conditions

	Cerebral Hemorrhage	Subarachnoid Hemorrhage	Brain Tumor	Multiple Sclerosis
Appearance	Bloody/xanthochromia	Bloody/xanthochromia	Clear/xanthochromia	Clear/colorless
Pressure	Normal	↑ (200–500)	↑ (200–500)	Normal
RBC	↑	↑	Normal to 50 lymph	Normal to 50 lymph

	↑ (45–100)	↑ (50–1000)	Normal to slightly ↑	Normal to 45–100
Protein				
Glucose	Normal	Normal	Normal to slightly ↓	Normal

Meningitis Finding in CSF

	Bacterial	Tuberculous	Viral/Aseptic	Fungal
Appearance	Turbid	Turbid	Clear/turbid	Variable
Pressure	↑ (200–500)	Variable	Normal	Variable
WBC (mm^3)	≥1000	Variable	<1000	Variable
WBC differential	PMNs	Lymphocytes	Lymphocytes	Lymphocytes
Protein (mg/dL)	↑ (50–500)	↑ (10–300)	↑ (45–200)	↑ (10–300)
Lactate (mM)	↑ >3	<2 mM	2–3	>3
Glucose	Absent/very low	<40	Normal	Low
CSF: glucose	Normal to marked ↑	↓	Usually normal	↓

TABLE 9–14: Seizure/Convulsion-like Activity

1. Assess patient and check vitals

2. Check meds that can ↓ seizure threshold: Levaquin, Wellbutrin, Synthroid, Amphetamines

3. If patient is on antiseizure meds → check level

4. BMP, Ca level, Mg level, Tox screen, ETOH level, UA, Blood C&S

5. ABG if patient appears cyanotic and check O_2 saturation

6. Check blood glucose (BGM) → low (<55) → thiamine 10 mg IV + 1 amp of $D_{50}W$ (1 amp can ↑ glucose level by 100)

7. Management → Bite block

- Diazepam 5 mg/min IV (0.2 mg/kg [max: 20 mg]) or

- Ativan 2 mg/min IV (0.1 mg/kg)

- Fosphenytoin 1000–1500 (15–20 mg/kg) IV in saline or dextrose solution at 150 mg/min or

- Phenytoin 15–20 mg/kg in 100 mL NS → give loading dose of 25–50 mg/min (max 1.5 g)

Note: Do not mix phenytoin with dextrose solution, if hypotension, reduce infusion rate.

- If seizure still persists → start phenobarbital 120–260 mg IV (10–20 mg/kg)

- If seizure continues → induce coma → propofol 1–2 mg/kg IV bolus then 2–4 mg/kg infusion or

TABLE 9–14 (Continued)

- Phenobarbital 10–15 mg/kg IV over 1–2 h then
  0.5–4 mg/kg/h infusion or

- Midazolam 0.2 mg/kg IV slowly followed by
  0.75–10 µg/kg/min infusion

Note: Patient needs intubation and ventilatory support, may
need vasopressor for hypotension

Note

- Fosphenytoin loading dose for seizure 15–20 mg/kg

- Phenytoin loading dose for seizure 15–20 mg/kg

- Correct phenytoin (Dilantin) for low albumin = measured
  dilantin/(albumin × 0.2) + 0.1

- Correct phenytoin (Dilantin) in renal failure = measured
  dilantin/(albumin × 0.1) + 0.1

TABLE 9–15: NIH Stroke Scale

Description	Score	Description	Score
Level of consciousness		**Motor upper extremity** (arms outstretched at 90° (sitting) or 45° (supine) × 10 s)	
Alert and responsive	0		
Arousable to minor stimuli	1	No drift	0
Arousable to only pain stimuli	2	Drift but does not fall to bed	1
Unarousable/reflex responses	3	Some antigravity but can't sustain	2
		No antigravity but some movement	3
Orientation			
Patient's name and current month	0	No movement	4
Patient's name or current month	1	**Motor lower extremity** (legs outstretched at 90° (sitting) or 45° (supine) × 10 s)	
Unable to state name or month	2		
Commands		No drift	0
Open and close eye and grip and release grip	0	Drift but does not fall to bed	1
Either of the two command	1	Some antigravity but can't sustain	2
Neither of the two command	2	No antigravity but some movement	3

TABLE 9–15 (Continued)			
Gaze (horizontal EOM by voluntary or Doll's eye)		No movement	4
		Limb ataxia, finger to nose and heel to shin	
Normal	0	No ataxia	0
Partial palsy	1	Ataxia in arms or legs	1
Forced eye deviation or total paresis	2	Ataxia in arms and legs	2
Visual field		**Sensory (test with sharp object)**	
Normal	0	Normal	0
Quadrantanopia	1	Unilateral loss but aware of touch	1
Hemianopia	2	Total unilateral loss	2
Blindness	3	Bilateral loss	3
Facial palsy (if stuporous check grimace)		**Language**	
Normal	0	Normal	0
Flat nasolabial fold, asymmetric smile	1	Moderate aphasia	1

(continued)

TABLE 9–15 (Continued)			
Lower face paralysis (partial)	2	Severe aphasia	2
Complete paralysis	3	Mute	3
Neglect (touch patient on both hands simultaneously, show fingers in both visual fields)		**Dysarthria (read set of words)**	
No neglect	0	Normal	0
Partial neglect (neglect in any modality)	1	Mild–moderate slurring	1
Total neglect (more than 1 modality)	2	Unintelligible or mute	2

TABLE 9–16: NIH Stroke Scale Score and Percent with Favorable Outcome

Score Age < 60 years	Percent with Favorable Outcome	Score Age 69–75 years	Percent with Favorable Outcome
0–9	42	0–9	54
10–14	18	10–14	27
15–20	27	15–20	0
>20	12	> 20	0
Age 61–68 years		**Age > 75 years**	
0–9	37	0–9	36
10–14	25	10–14	15
15–20	25	15–20	6
>20	0	>20	0

Source with permission: NINDS t-PA stroke study group, National Institute of Health (NIH).

TABLE 9–17: Stroke Management

1. Assess patient

2. Search for risk factors for stroke

3. Monitor vitals, pulse ox, and ECG

4. Check blood glucose (BGM), CBC with diff, platelet, BMP, PT, PTT, INR, EKG, CX Ray

5. Head CT (noncontrast)

6. MRI is better if very small stroke is suspected or lesion is noted to be in brain stem

MRI contraindications: see below

7. Start aspirin 325 mg PO daily ± clopidogrel (Plavix) 75 mg PO daily if CT/MRI is (−) for bleed (hemorrhagic stroke)

   • Aggrenox (ASA + dipyridamole) 1 tab PO bid has been shown to be more effective than aspirin for prevention of stroke

   • Alternative drug that can be used is ticlopidine 250 mg bid but its side effects are neutropenia, thrombocytopenia

8. rt-PA can be used in non-hemorrhagic stroke and should present within 3 hrs, recommended by NINDS (National Institute of Neurological Disorders and Stroke). See: exclusion criteria below

   • rt-PA: 0.9 mg/kg (max: 90 mg) 10% IV bolus and then give 90% over 1 h infusion

   • Do not give ASA, heparin, or warfarin during 1st 24 h if rt-PA is given

9. Heparin and warfarin use in atherosclerotic stroke is controversial

TABLE 9–17 (Continued)

10. Heparin and warfarin are indicated in patient with cardiogenic emboli (keep INR = 2–3, 2.5–3.5 in mechanical valve). See exclusion criteria below for starting patient on heparin and warfarin

11. BP management: lowering BP in acute cerebral infarction setting is contraindicated unless following:

BP: Sys > 230 or Dia > 120	Hypertensive encephalopathy is present
Vital organs are compromised due to BP	Cerebral ischemia 2° to aortic dissection

12. DVT prophylaxis: if patient is not receiving heparin/warfarin/rt-PA → place patient on SCD or heparin 5000 units Sub Q bid–tid

13. Keep NPO until swallowing evaluation is performed

14. Consults: neurology, speech, physical therapy, and occupational therapy

15. Studies to consider

Carotid duplex US	Cardiac ECHO		Holter	Lipid profile
ESR	ANA	Protein C and S		Anticardiolipin antibody
Lupus anticoagulant		Coagulation panel		Hemoglobin electrophoresis

Note: If Patient placed on Lovenox → check antifactor Xa after 4–6 h after the 1st dose.

(continued)

TABLE 9–17 (Continued)

rt-PA Inclusion Criteria in Patient with Stroke

1. Age > 18 years

2. Clinical evidence of ischemic stroke with neurological deficit

3. Time of onset < 3 h

rt-PA Exclusion criteria in patient with stroke

Historical relevance

1. Stroke or head trauma within past 3 months

2. Prior history of intracranial hemorrhage

3. Any major surgery within past 14 days

4. GI or GU bleeding within past 21 days

5. MI in past 3 months

6. Arterial puncture at non-compressible site within past 7 days

7. Lumbar puncture within past 7 days

Clinical relevance

8. Rapidly improving symptoms of stroke

9. Isolated or minor neurologic signs

10. Seizure at onset of stroke with post-ictal residual impairments

11. Symptoms suggestive of subarachnoid hemorrhage (with negative head CT)

TABLE 9–17 (Continued)

12. Presentation consistent with acute MI or post-MI pericarditis

13. Persistent BP Systolic >185, Diastolic >110

14. Pregnancy/Lactation

15. Active bleeding

Relevance of lab

16. Platelets <100,000/mm^3

17. Glucose <50 mg/dl (2.8 mmol/L) or >400 mg/dl (22.3 mmol/L)

18. INR > 1.7 if on coumadin

19. Elevated PTT if on Heparin

Relevance of Radiologic studies

20. Head CT shows evidence of hemorrhage

21. Head CT shows early infarct signs (diffuse swelling, parenchymal hypodensity, and/or effacement of >33% of middle cerebral artery territory

Source with permission: Report of quality standard subcommittee of American Academy of Neurology. Neurology, Sep 1996; 47:835–839

(continued)

TABLE 9–17 (Continued)

Heparin and Warfarin Exclusion Criteria in Patient with Stroke

1. CT/MRI scan shows: hemorrhage, tumor, abscess, epidural or subdural hematoma

2. Current bleeding

3. History of GI bleeding, bleeding tendencies

4. Large infarction noted on CT/MRI scan

5. Neurological deterioration secondary to severe cerebral edema

6. Recent surgery past 14 days

7. Severe uncontrolled hypertension (BP > 185/110)

MRI Contraindications

Cardiac pacemaker	Implanted cardiac defibrillator
Aneurysm clips	Carotid artery vascular clamp
Neurostimulator	Implanted drug infusion device
Bone growth/fusion stimulator	Cochlear, otologic, or ear implant
Metallic splinters in eye	Hemostatic CNS clips

TABLE 9–18: Bell's Palsy

Signs and Symptoms

- May start with eye itching and lacrimation

- Abnormal taste (metallic)

- Unilateral face weakness including upper face (eyebrow orbicularis weakness) and lower face (Nasolabial fold)

- Pain or pressure behind ear

- Hyperacusis

Tests to Consider

CBC with diff	ESR	CX Ray (R/O TB, sarcoid, adenopathy)
ACE level (for sarcoid)	HIV	MRI/CT
EMG (electro-myogram)	EnoG (electro-neurography)	EEMG (evoked electromyogram)
Urine Bence Jones protein (in elderly)		Serum immuno-electrophoresis (in elderly)

(continued)

TABLE 9–18 (Continued)
Therapy
• Supportive
• Artificial tears (Akwa Tears, AquaSite, Bion, Isopto, Liquifilm, Moisture)
• Eye protection (protective glasses or goggles during day and patch at night)
• Oral[a] prednisone 1 mg/kg/day × 7 days (best if used within 24 h)
• (Be cautious of using steroid in patient with diabetes, peptic ulcer disease, renal or hepatic dysfunction or severe hypertension)
• Valacyclovir[a] (1 g PO bid–tid × 7 days or famciclovir 750 mg PO tid)
[a]A report of the Quality Standards Subcommittee of the American Academy of Neurology concluded that an advantage from steroids and acyclovir has not been definitively recognized in patients with Bell's palsy.
Note: Central lesion spares paralysis of forehead muscles.

TABLE 9–19: Guillain-Barré Syndrome (Acute Idiopathic Demyelinating Polyradiculoneuritis)

Signs and Symptoms	Therapy
• Poor breathing and swallowing	• Intubate if respiratory depression
• Stocking and glove numbness of hands and feet	• Plasmapheresis
• Rapid symmetric weakness	• IV Immunoglobulin
• Weak DTRs	• Eye drops for drying eyes
• Facial diplegia	• Narcotics can be useful for back pain
• Diffuse back pain	• Supportive care

TABLE 9–20: Vertigo

Central	Peripheral
• Chronic onset (if sudden, with headache)	• Often sudden onset
• Usually not associated with hearing loss	• Associated with hearing loss or tinnitus
• Symptoms independent of position	• Symptoms associated with position
• Absence of tinnitus	• Tinnitus may be present
• Nausea	• Usually severe nausea
• Severe instability	• Unidirectional instability
• Nausea	• Usually severe nausea
• Vertical nystagmus (very specific)	• May have rotatory or horizontal nystagmus
• Falling to the same side of lesion	• Falling to the opposite side of lesion

Etiology	
Central	Peripheral
• Brainstem lesion	• Benign positional vertigo
• Cerebellar lesion/disease	• Méniere's disease
• Neuroma	• Vestibular neuronitis
• Transient ischemic attacks (TIAs)	• Infection: otitis media, zoster, syphilis
• Meds: phenytoin or barbiturates	• Meds: furosemide, quinine, quinidine, ASA, antibiotics, ETOH

TABLE 9–20 (Continued)

Management of Vertigo

- Diphenhydramine 10–50 mg IM/IV q4-6 (useful for acute management) or

- Prochlorperazine 5–10 mg IM/IV q6h or

- Meclizine 25–50 mg PO q6h or

- Dimenhydrinate 50 mg PO q4-6h or

- Scopolamine 1 patch q3h or

- Diazepam 5–10 mg PO q12h or

- Lorazepam 1–2 mg PO q8h

10
Psychiatry

TABLE 10–1: DSM IV Axis Classifications of Diagnosis

Axis I	Clinical psychiatric disorders (e.g., major depressive disorder, bipolar disorders, schizophrenia)
Axis II	Personality disorders/mental retardation
Axis III	General medical condition that may be relevant in understanding psych condition
Axis IV	Psychosocial stressors (divorce, death of a family member, trip, loss of job)
Axis V	Defined according to global assessment functioning scale (scale rates psychological, social, and occupational functioning on a hypothetical continuum on mental health illness)

TABLE 10–2: Assessment of Mental Status

Appearance: well groomed, disheveled, relaxed

Motor: tics, tremors, lethargic, dystonia, activity

Speech: slow, fast, paused, dysarthric

Thought content: delusions, persecutions, obsessions

Thought form: loose, circumstantial, logical

Affect: flat, excited, jovial (your own observation)

Mood: depressed, euphoric, labile (patient's feelings reported)

Insight: good, fair, poor (patient's understanding of his condition)

Judgment: good, fair, poor (patient's ability to make decisions)

TABLE 10–3: Mini-Cog (Dementia Screening)

1. Registration: tell patient 3 objects (car, pen, and shirt); ask to repeat and remember them

2. Clock drawing: ask patient to draw a clock and have him place the clock hands at 11:20

3. Recall: ask patient to recall the 3 objects that you asked him to remember

Interpretation

- Patient is unable to recall any of the 3 objects: dementia highly likely

- Patient is able to recall all 3 objects: dementia unlikely

- Patient is able to recall 1 or 2 objects and clock is abnormal: dementia highly likely

- Patient is able to recall 1 or 2 objects and clock is normal: dementia unlikely

Source with permission: Mini-Cog™ copyright 2000, 2003, 2005 by Dr. Soo Borson and James Soley. All rights reserved. Reprinted under license from University of Washington solely for use as clinical or teaching aid. Any other use is strictly prohibited without permission from Dr. Borson, soob@u.washington.edu

TABLE 10–4: Major Depressive Disorder

Patient have >5 symptoms for >2 weeks, at least one of these symptoms MUST be either (1) depressed mood or (2) loss of interest/pleasure

1. Depressed mood most of the day, nearly everyday. (Children and elderly may show irritability)

2. Anhedonia (low interest or pleasure in most activities most of the day, nearly everyday)

3. Significant weight loss or gain (significant ↑ or ↓ in appetite)

4. Insomnia or hypersomnia

5. Psychomotor agitation or psychomotor retardation

6. Fatigue or loss of energy

7. Feeling of worthlessness or guilt

8. Decreased ability to concentrate

9. Recurrent thoughts of death, recurrent suicidal ideation

TABLE 10–5: Geriatric Depression Scale (GDS) Score	
1. Are you basically satisfied with your life?	Yes/**No**
2. Have you dropped many of your activities and interests?	**Yes**/No
3. Do you feel that your life is empty?	**Yes**/No
4. Do you often get bored?	**Yes**/No
5. Are you in good spirit most of the time?	Yes/**No**
6. Are you afraid that something bad is going to happen to you?	**Yes**/No
7. Do you feel happy most of the time?	Yes/**No**
8. Do you often feel helpless?	**Yes**/No
9. Do you prefer to stay at home, rather than going out and doing new things?	**Yes**/No
10. Do you feel you have more problems with memory than most?	**Yes**/No
11. Do you think it is wonderful to be alive now?	Yes/**No**
12. Do you feel pretty worthless the way you are now?	**Yes**/No
13. Do you feel full of energy?	Yes/**No**
14. Do you feel that your situation is hopeless?	**Yes**/No
15. Do you feel that most people are better off than you are?	**Yes**/No
Score: >5 bold answers checked → suggests depression	

Reproduced with permission: Sheikh JI, Yasavage JA, Brink TL. Recent evidence and development of short version. *Clinical Gerontol* 1986;5:165.

TABLE 10–6: Manic Episode

>1 week of abnormally and persistently elevated, expansive, irritable mood plus ≥ 3 of below:

1. Elevated self-esteem or grandiosity

2. Decreased need for sleep

3. Pressured speech

4. Flight of ideas (jumping rapidly from one thought to another)

5. Increased distractibility

6. Psychomotor agitation or goal-directed behavior

7. Involved in a pleasurable activities that have bad consequences (e.g., gambling, unprotected sex, IVDA)

TABLE 10–7: Delirium vs. Dementia

Delirium	Dementia
Rapid onset (hour to day)	Gradual onset (month to year)
Fluctuating altered level of consciousness	Normal level of consciousness
↓ Awareness of environment (poor attention)	Attention is usually intact
↓ Ability to concentrate	Memory deficit
Memory deficit	Language disturbance
Hallucinations	Apraxia
Language disturbance	Agnosia
Etiology: meds, toxin, illness	Etiology: Alzheimer's, multi-infarct, HIV/AIDS

TABLE 10–8: Alcohol Abuse Screening (CAGE)

1. Cut down (Have you ever felt the need to cutdown on drinking?)

2. Annoyed (Have you ever been annoyed by family/friends nagging you about drinking?)

3. Guilty (Have you ever felt guilty about drinking?)

4. Eyeopener (Have you ever had an eye-opener [Need to drink first thing in the morning?])

11
Pulmonary Disease

FIGURE 11–1: PA CX Ray Landmarks/Lateral CX Ray Landmarks

PA Cxray Landmarks			Lateral Cxray Landmarks		

1	SVC	A	® LL	1	Posterior clear space	A	Right/left lower lobe
2	® Atrium	B	® ML	2	Anterior clear space	B	Right middle lobe or lingular segment Ⓛ
3	® Ventricle	C	Lingular segment	3	Ⓛ Ventricle	R	Right hilum
4	Ⓛ Ventricle	D	Ⓛ Lower lobe	4	Ⓛ Atrium	L	Left hilum
5	Ⓛ Atrium						
6	Aortic knob						

Copyright: Anil Patel, MD

TABLE 11–1: Note

- Steroids are useful in COPD (chronic obstructive pulmonary disease) patient (Solu-Medrol 60–80 mg IV q6-8h)

- Indication for home O_2 is

  1. $PaO_2 < 55$ or O_2 saturation $< 88\%$

  2. $PaO_2 <55$–59 or O_2 saturation <88–89% and Cor pulmonale or polycythemia

- ΔCO_2 of 10 ΔpH by 0.08

- Patient with COPD are usually CO_2 and HCO_3 retainers

- A-a gradient = $[(713 \times FiO_2) - (PaCO_2/0.8)] - PaO_2$

- $PaCO_2$ (arterial CO_2 tension) = 35–44 mmHg

- $PACO_2$ (alveolar CO_2 tension) = 40 mmHg

- Nasal cannula can give maximum O_2 of 6 L

- If > 6 L is required → must use high flow NC (nasal cannula)

- When using O_2 > 4 L → should use humidifier

TABLE 11–2: Normal Pulmonary Function Test

FEV1	FVC	FEV1/FVC	FEF 25–50	MVV
40 mL/kg	30–50 mL/kg	>85%	3–4 L/s	>150 L/min
TLC (total lung capacity) = 4–6 L			VC (vital capacity) = 3–5 L	
TV (tidal volume) = 7–10 mL/kg		RV (residual volume) = 1–2.4 L		
FEV = forced expiratory volume		FEF = forced expiratory flow		
FVC = forced vital capacity		MVV = maximal voluntary ventilation		

FIGURE 11–2: Normal Pulmonary Function Test

Maximal inspiration

TLC = Total lung capacity
VC = Vital capacity
RV = Residual volume
IC = Inspiratory capacity
FRC = Functional residual capacity
IRV = Inspiratory reserve volume
TV = Tidal volume (Normal inspiration and expiration)
ERV = Expiratory reserve volume

Maximal expiration

TABLE 11–2 (Continued)						
Pulmonary Function Test Interpretation (PFT)						
Condition	FEV1	FVC	FEV1/ FVC	RV	TLC	DLCO
Obstruction	↓	N/↓	↓	N/↑	N/↑	N/↓
Restriction (extrinsic)	N/↓	↓	N/↑	N/↓	↓	N
Restriction (intrinsic)	N/↓	↓	N/↑	N/↓	↓	↓
Combined (obstruction + restriction)	↓	↓	↓	N/↓	↓	N/↓

Note: DLCO is normal in bronchitis but decreased in emphysema, may be ↑ in asthma.

TABLE 11–3: Pleural Fluid Analysis

Fluid	Transudate	Exudate	Transudate	Exudate
Protein	<3 g/dL	>3 g/dL	CHF	PE, pulmonary infarction
LDH	<200 U/L	>200 U/L	Cirrhosis	Infection/TB
SG	<1.016	>1.016	Nephrotic syndrome	Malignancy
Fluid:serum protein ratio	<0.5	>0.5	Hypoalbumin	Collagen vascular disease
			Glomerulonephritis	Esophageal rupture/trauma
Fluid:serum LDH ratio	<0.6	>0.6	Constrictive pericarditis	Hypothyroidism
			Atelectasis	Pancreatitis

Note

- The following are exudates that can present as transudates—malignancy, PE, sarcoid.
- The following is a transudate that can present as exudates—CHF.
- Hemothorax: pleural fluid Hct:serum Hct ratio → >0.5 (50%).
- Chylothorax: TG > 110 mg/dL.
- If pleural fluid pH < 7.2 → may have possible empyema.

TABLE 11–4: Well's Criteria for Pulmonary Embolism (Modified)	
Criteria	**Score**
Clinical symptoms of DVT	3
Other diagnosis less likely than PE	3
Heart rate > 100	1.5
Immobilization or surgery in past 4 weeks	1.5
Previous DVT/PE	1.5
Hemoptysis	1
Malignancy	1

Score	Probability of Patient Having PE
<2	Low
2–6	Moderate
>6	High

Source: With permission from Dr. Philip Wells.

Common Etiologies for PE		
Immobilization	Malignancy	Surgery within past 3 months
Factor V Leiden	History of thromboembolism	
OCP (oral contraceptive) use	Hypercoagulable state	

(continued)

TABLE 11–4 (Continued)		
Labs/Studies in PE		
CBC	BMP	PT/PTT/INR
ABG	Troponin	Spiral CT (be cautious in patient with renal failure)
V/Q scan	CXR PA and lateral	Anticardiolipin antibody
Protein C&S	Quantitative D-dimer	Venous Doppler (lower extremity)
Fibrinogen	ECG	Antithrombin III deficiency
Stool guaiac	Pulmonary angiogram	Impedance plethysmography (lower extremity)
Meds: Pulmonary Embolism		
1. Heparin: bolus 80 unit/kg IV → then 18 unit/kg/h, √ PTT 6 h after starting infusion (keep PTT 1.5–2 CTRL) or Lovenox 1 mg/kg Sub Q q12h or 1.5 mg/kg Sub Q daily		
2. Start warfarin 5–10 mg PO daily (maintain INR 2–3) when PTT becomes therapeutic		

TABLE 11–4 (Continued)

3. Pulmonary embolectomy or thrombolytics [alteplase/ streptokinase (check fibrinogen before starting)] if patient develops hypotension requiring vasopressor and has documented PE with angiography

   - Alteplase 100 mg IV over 2 h → then heparin infusion 15 unit/kg/h (keep PTT 1.5–2 CTRL) or streptokinase 250,000 units IV over 30 min → then 100,000 unit/h × 24–72 h → then heparin infusion 15 unit/kg/h (keep PTT 1.5–2 CTRL)

4. IVC filter: indicated in patient who has contraindication to anticoagulant or recurrent PE

5. Meperidine 25–100 mg IV prn for pain

6. Ranitidine 150 mg PO bid prn

TABLE 11–5: Asthma Classification and Management

Asthma Classification

Category	Days with Symptom	Nights with Symptom	FEV1/PEF	PEF Variability
Mild intermittent	≤2/weeks	≤2/months	≥80%	<20%
Mild persistent	>2/weeks	>2/months	≥80%	20–30%
Moderate persistent	Daily	>1/week	60–80%	>30%
Severe persistent	Continuous	Frequent	≤60%	>30%

Asthma Management

Category	Rescue Medication	Control Medication
Mild intermittent	Short β_2 agonist	None
Mild persistent	Short β_2 agonist	1st Line: inhaled corticosteroid (Low dose)
		2nd Line: cromolyn, leukotriene inhibitor, theophylline

Moderate persistent	Short β_2 agonist	1st Line: inhaled corticosteroid (low–medium dose) + long-acting inhaled β_2 agonist
		2nd Line: add leukotriene or theophylline to inhaled β_2 corticosteroid (low–medium dose)
Severe persistent	Short β_2 agonist	1st Line: inhaled corticosteroid (high dose) + long-acting inhaled β_2 agonist
		2nd Line: inhaled corticosteroid (high dose) + long-acting inhaled β_2 agonist + systemic corticosteroids

Source with permission: Expert panel report II: Guidelines for the diagnosis and management of asthma. Feb. 1997, and update on selected topics 2002; NAEPP expert panel report II (NIH publication, National Heart, Lung, and Blood Institute, NHLBI guidelines).

(continued)

TABLE 11–5 (Continued)

Asthma (Exacerbation) Management

1. Oxygenation to achieve sat of at least > 90%

2. β_2 Agonist (short) → albuterol 2.5 mg via nebulizer q20 min or 6–12 puffs via MDI

   → Severe → albuterol 2.5–5 mg with Ipratropium 0.5 mg via nebulizer

   → Albuterol 10–15 mg nebulizer over 1 h

3. Check pre- and posttherapy peak flow

4. Methylprednisolone 125 mg IV initially then 40–60 mg IV q6h then to PO prednisone 60 mg q6-8h then taper

5. If all above fails → consider epinephrine 0.3 mL of a 1:1000 Sub Q q20min × 3 doses

   → Terbutaline 0.25 mg Sub Q q6-8h

6. If infection is suspected → consider using antibiotics

Note: If patient develops tachycardia/palpitation/tremors → use Xopenex 0.63–1.25 mg q6-8.

TABLE 11–6: Long-term Control Medication for Asthma		
Medication	**≤12 Years**	**>12 Years**
Inhaled corticosteroids (see table below)		
Long-acting inhaled β_2 agonist		
• Salmeterol MDI 21 µg/puff	1–2 puffs q12h	2 puffs q12h
• Salmeterol DPI 50 µg/blister	1 blister q12h	1 blister q12h
• Formoterol DPI 12 µg/single-use capsule	1 capsule q12h	1 capsule q12h
Combined medication (steroid and β_2 agonist)		
• Fluticasone + salmeterol DPI (100, 250, and 500 µg/50 µg)	1 inhale bid	1 inhale bid
Cromolyn MDI 1 mg/puff	1–2 puffs tid–qid	1 puffs bid–tid
Cromolyn nebulizer 20 mg/ampule	1 ampule tid–qid	1 ampule tid–qid
Nedocromil MDI 1.75 mg/puff	1–2 puffs bid–qid	2–4 puffs bid–qid

(continued)

TABLE 11–6 (Continued)		
Leukotriene modifiers		
• Montelukast 4, 5, 10 mg chewable tablets	4 mg qhs (2–5 years)	10 mg qhs
	5 mg qhs (6–14 years)	
	10 mg qhs (>14 years)	
• Zafirlukast 10, 20 mg tablet	10 mg bid (7–11 years)	20 mg bid
• Zileuton 300, 600 mg	X	600 mg qid
Methylxanthine (Theophylline)		
• Sustained release tablet, liquid, capsule • Starting dose 10 mg/kg/day up to 300 mg	<1 year: $0.2 \times$ (age in weeks) + 5 = mg/kg/day	Usual max: 800 mg/day
	≥1 year: 16 mg/kg/day	

TABLE 11–7: GOLDS Criteria for Disease Severity in COPD Patient

0—At risk	• Normal spirometry • Chronic symptoms (cough, sputum)
I—Mild	• FEV/FVC < 70% • FEV ≥ 80% predicted with or without symptoms
II—Moderate	• FEV/FVC < 70% • FEV < 80% or >50% predicted with or without chronic symptoms
III—Severe	• FEV/FVC < 70% • FEV < 50% or >30% predicted with or without chronic symptoms
IV—Very severe	• FEV/FVC < 70% • FEV < 30% predicted

Reprinted with permission: Calverley MA, Walker P. Chronic obstructive pulmonary disease. *Lancet* 2003;362:1053–1061.

TABLE 11–8: Treatment Modalities for GOLDS Stages for Patient with COPD

GOLDS Stages	First Line	Second Line

0–I	• Risk factor avoidance
	  Smoking cessation
	  Influenza vaccine
		• Short-acting bronchodilator prn

II	• As stage I + add long-acting bronchodilators, preferably inhaled	• Pulmonary rehabilitation
III	• As stage II + add long-acting inhaled corticosteroids	• Pulmonary rehabilitation
IV	• As stage III + add long-acting domiciliary oxygen	• If respiratory failure → surgery

Reprinted with permission: Calverley MA, Walker P. Chronic obstructive pulmonary disease. *Lancet* 2003;362:1053–1061.

Chr. cough
sputum
wheezing
dyspnea

Stable COPD : smoking cessation
long act Bronchodilators (B-A/anti dhol)
& or inhaled corticosteroids
Vaccine: influenza pneumoc.pneu
pulmonary rehab
oxygen therapy

$FEV_1 < 60\%$ – criterion for pharmacol. therapy
$FEV_1 < 50\%$ consider pulm rehab.

TABLE 11–9: Management of Exacerbation of COPD

Search for Underlying Etiology for Exacerbation and Treat the Cause

1. Oxygenation to achieve sat of at least 89–90% $PO_2 \leq 55$ or $SpO_2 \leq 88\%$ (start with 2 L NC, a high oxygen content can suppress their CO_2 drive thus avoid high oxygenation).
   - A higher requirement means worsening condition

2. Breathing Rx with β agonist is essential (e.g., albuterol, Duoneb [albuterol + ipratropium])
   Note: If tachycardia occurs with β agonist agents, consider Xopenex.

3. Inhaled bronchodilators such as albuterol, metaproterenol, or terbutaline 2–4 puffs q30-60min then ↓ to 2–4 puffs q3-4h

4. Ipratropium 4–6 puffs q4-6h

5. Methylprednisolone 125 mg IV initially then ↓ to 60–100 mg IV q6-8h
   Note: Change to oral prednisone 40–60 mg PO daily after 2–3days if the patient's COPD is stable.

6. Theophylline 5 mg/kg IV bolus over 20 min, then 400–600 mg PO daily. Giving theophylline is controversial
   Note: Therapeutic range is 8–12 mg/dL. Theophylline may cause tachyarrhythmia.

7. Guaifenesin 100–400 mg PO q4-6h for cough and clearance of the secretion

8. If respiratory infection is suspected → consider
   → TMP–SMX DS 1 tab PO bid or
   → Amoxicillin 250 mg PO tid or
   → Doxycycline 100 mg PO bid or
   → Azithromycin 500 mg PO on day 1 and 250 mg PO daily day 2–5

12
Rheumatology

TABLE 12–1: Crystal-induced Arthritis

Gout	Pseudogout
• Monosodium urate crystals	• Calcium pyrophosphate dihydrate crystal
• Negatively birefringent	• Weakly positive birefringent
• Needle-shaped crystals	• Linear or rhomboid-shaped crystals
• Monoarticular > oligoarticular	• Monoarticular > oligoarticular

Acute Rx treatment options for gout and pseudogout

1. Indomethacin 25–50 mg PO q6h × 2 days then, 50 mg tid × 2 days, then 25 mg tid (1st line)

2. Toradol (ketorolac) 30–60 mg IM, then 15–30 mg IM q6h/10 mg PO tid–qid (2nd line) or

3. Ibuprofen 800 mg, then 400–800 PO q4-6h

TABLE 12–1 (Continued)

4. Methylprednisone 125 mg IV × 1 dose then prednisone 40–60 mg PO daily/5days → taper

5. Colchicine 0.5–0.6 mg PO 2 tab followed by 1 tab qh until relief (max dose of 9.6 mg/24 h) then 0.5–0.6 PO daily–bid

6. Pain management: Meperidine 50–100 mg IM/IV q4-6h prn

Chronic management of Hyperuricemia

Allopurinol 300 mg PO daily, may ↑ to 100–300 mg q2week or

Probenecid 250 mg PO bid, ↑ 500 mg bid after 1 week, then ↑ by 500 mg q4week

TABLE 12–2: Giant Cell Arteritis

History

• Headache	• Anorexia/weight loss
• Jaw/tongue claudication	• Visual disturbance
• Arthralgia/arthritis	• Myalgia

Physical Examination

- Temporal artery tenderness, erythema, swollen, and warm
- Visual disturbance
- TIA/stroke
- Scalp tenderness

Labs/Studies

• CBC with diff	• ESR
• Temporal artery biopsy	• Alkaline phosphatase
• Temporal arteriography	• AST

Treatment

Corticosteroid IV initially then → switch to PO steroids

TABLE 12–3: Synovial Fluid Analysis

	Septic	Inflammatory	Noninflammatory	Hemorrhagic
Color	Yellow-green	Yellow	Yellow	Red
Viscosity	Variable	Low	High	Variable
WBC/mm³	>75K	25–50K	<10K	<10K
PMNs (%)	>75	>50	<25	50–75
Glucose (mg/dL)	<25	>25	Equal to serum	Equal to serum
Protein (g/dL)	3–5	3–5	1–3	4–6

TABLE 12–4: Antibodies and their Clinical Significance

Antibodies	Clinical Significance
Antiacetylcholine receptor	Myasthenia gravis
Anticardiolipin	Positive in SLE (associated with thrombosis and fetal loss), (+)
	May be positive in some autoimmune disease
Anticentromere	CREST syndrome of scleroderma, Raynaud's disease, Sjögren's syndrome, SLE
Anti-DNase-B	Streptococcal pyodermal infection and acute glomerulonephritis
	Postimpetigo nephritis
Anti-DS DNA	Specific for SLE
Antigliadin	Celiac disease
Antiglomerular basement	Goodpasture's syndrome
Antihistone	Positive in drug-associated SLE
Antimitochondrial	Primary biliary cirrhosis
Antinuclear	Sensitive for SLE, may be (+) in autoimmune and inflammatory dz.

TABLE 12–4 (Continued)	
Antinucleolar, SCL-70	Progressive systemic sclerosis
ANCA (antineutrophilic cytophilic antibodies)	Wegener's granulomatosis, microscopic polyarteritis
	Churg-Strauss syndrome, polyarteritis nodosum
Anti-RANA	Rheumatoid arthritis
Antiribonucleoprotein	Mixed connective tissue disease
Anti-RO (SSA) and anti-La (SSB)	Positive in Sjögren's syndrome
Anti-Sm (Smith)	Specific for SLE
Antithyroglobulin or antimicrosomal	Hashimoto's thyroiditis
Lupus anticoagulant	Associated with thrombosis, fetal loss, and bleeding diathesis

13
Toxicology

TABLE 13–1: Life-threatening Poisoning

Hemodialysis can be Useful with Following Poisoning

• Ethylene glycol	• Salicylate
• Lithium	• Theophylline
• Methanol	

Charcoal Hemoperfusion can be Useful with Following Poisoning

• Theophylline	• Salicylate
• Phenobarbital	• Paraquat

TABLE 13–2: Poisoning Toxidrome

Stimulants	Depressants
• Anticholinergics	• Antidepressants
• Amphetamines	• Cholinergics
• Cocaine	• Narcotics
• Sedative withdrawal	• Sedatives

Signs and Symptoms

• Agitation	• Miosis
• Fever	• Mydriasis
• Hyperreflexia	• Respiratory depression
• Hypertension	• Seizure
• Hyporeflexia	• Sweating
• Lethargy → coma	• Tachycardia

TABLE 13–3: Poisoning (General Management)

1. Stabilize patient—ABCs

2. Consider elective intubation in comatose patient

3. Call poison control

4. IVF if patient is hypotensive

5. Oxygen

6. Thiamine

7. Glucose

8. Naloxone

9. Monitor: vital signs and mental status

The Following Drug Overdose Requires Level to Determine Severity of Overdose and Treatment Options

• Acetaminophen	• Ethylene glycol	• Methanol
• Arsenic	• Iron	• Salicylate
• Carbon monoxide	• Lead	• Theophylline
• Digoxin	• Lithium	

Activated charcoal is ineffective for the followings

- Alcohol

- Lithium

- Iron

- Absolute contraindications to charcoal are corrosives

TABLE 13–4: Acetaminophen Overdose (Toxic Dose: 7.5 g or >140 mg/kg)

Stage I (First 24 H)	Stage II (24–72 H)
• N/V	• ↑ LFT may be seen
• Diaphoresis	• Nephrotoxicity and pancreatitis may be seen
• Pallor	• Right upper quadrant pain and tenderness
• Lethargy/malaise	• ↑ PT, total bilirubin
• May be asymptomatic	• Oliguria
• LFT may be normal	• ↑ Amylase and lipase
Stage III (72–96 H)	**Stage IV (4 Days to 2 Weeks)**
• ↑ LFT (LFT peaks)	• Recovery is slower in this phase
• Jaundice	• All labs may not normalize for several weeks
• Confusion (2° to hepatic encephalopathy)	• ↑ LFT
• ↑ Ammonia	• Jaundice
• ↑ PT, total bilirubin	• Confusion (2° to hepatic encephalopathy)
• Hypoglycemia	• ↑ Ammonia
• Lactic acidosis	• ↑ PT, total bilirubin

TABLE 13–4 (Continued)	
• Acute renal failure (2° to ATN)	• Hypoglycemia
	• Lactic acidosis
	• Acute renal failure (2° to ATN)

Note: Alcoholics, malnourished, and patients on anticonvulsants are more prone to liver injury at smaller doses.

Management of Adverse Reaction to IV *N*-Acetylcysteine (NAC)

Reaction	Rx for Adult	Rx for Pediatric
1. Flushing	Continue without NAC treatment	Continue NAC without treatment
2. Urticaria	Diphenhydramine 50 mg IV	1 mg/kg up to 50 mg
3. Angioedema	D/C NAC→ diphenhydramine	D/C NAC → diphenhydramine
	50 mg IV and restart NAC at slower	→ 1 mg/kg up to 50 mg
	rate in 1 h if symptoms resolve	and restart NAC at slower rate in
		1 h if symptoms resolve

(continued)

TABLE 13–4 (Continued)		
4. Wheezing	D/C NAC → give supportive care	D/C NAC → give supportive care
or	Diphenhydramine 50 mg IV	Diphenhydramine → 1 mg/kg max 50 mg
Hypotension	Consider decreasing infusion rate	Consider decreasing infusion rate
	Consider ranitidine 50 mg IV	Consider ranitidine IV 1 mg/kg up to 50 mg
	Consider epinephrine (1:1000)	Consider epinephrine (1:1000)
	0.3–0.5 mL Sub Q consider fluids	0.1 mg/kg consider fluids
	Restart NAC IV at slower rate in 1 h	Restart NAC IV at slower rate in 1 h
	if symptoms resolve/change PO	if symptoms resolve or change to oral

Source with permission: Bailey B, McGuigan MA. Management of anaphylactoid reaction to IV N-acetylcysteine. *Ann Emerg Med* 1998;31:710–715, American College of Emergency Physicians.

TABLE 13–4 (Continued)	
Management	
• Lavage	
• Activated charcoal	
• *N*-Acetylcysteine using above nomogram (best if used within 8 h)	
• Use *N*-Acetyl protocol for further management:	
1. 72 h FDA approved protocol: PO only	
2. 48 h IV bolus protocol	
3. 20 h infusion protocol: IV	
72 H *N*-Acetylcysteine Oral Protocol	**20 H *N*-Acetylcysteine IV Protocol**
140 mg/kg loading dose	150 mg/kg over 1 h
70 mg/kg q4h × 68 h	50 mg/kg over 4 h or 12.5 mg/kg/h × 4 h
48 H *N*-Acetylcysteine IV Protocol	100 mg/kg over 16 h or 6.25 mg/kg/h
140 mg/kg loading dose	
70 mg/kg q4h × 12 h	

Source with permission: Prescott LF, Park J, Ballantyne A, et al. Treatment of paracetamol with N-acetylcysteine. *Lancet.* 1977;2:432–434; Smilkstein MJ, Bronstein AC, Linden C, et al. Acetaminophen overdose: A 48 hour *N*-acetylcysteine treatment protocol. *Ann Emerg Med.* 1991;20(10): 105–1063, American College of Emergency Physicians.

FIGURE 13–1: Relationship between Acetaminophen Overdose and Liver Toxicity

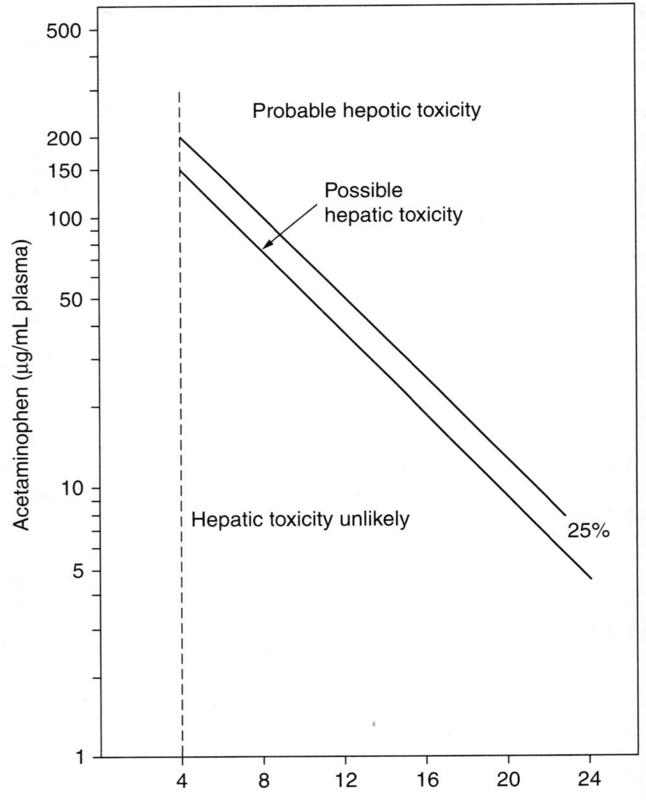

TABLE 13–5: Alcohol Withdrawal Symptoms

Time Elapsed After Last Drink	Clinical Finding Correlating with Time Elapsed After Last Drink	
• 6–36 h	• Anxiety	• GI upset
	• Anorexia	• Headache
	• Diaphoresis	• Tremulousness
• 6–48 h	• Generalized tonic–clonic seizure	• Status epilepticus
• 12–48 h	• Hallucinations—visual (occasionally auditory or tactile)	
• 48–96 h	• Agitation	• Fever
	• Delirium	• Hypertension
	• Diaphoresis	• Tachycardia

TABLE 13–6: Clinical Withdrawal Assessment Scale for Alcohol, Revised (CIWA–AR)

Score	Nausea and Vomiting	Headache	Paroxysmal Sweats
0	No nausea or vomiting	Not present	No sweat noted
1		Very mild	Barely perceptible
2		Mild	
3		Moderate	
4	Intermittent nausea with dry heaves	Moderately severe	Beads of sweat noted on forehead
5		Severe	
6		Very severe	
7	Constant N/V and dry heaves	Extremely severe	Drenching sweats
Score	Anxiety	Agitation	Tremor
0	No anxiety	No agitation	No tremor
1		More than normal activity	Tremor can be felt at fingertip
2			
3			

TABLE 13–6 (Continued)			
4	Moderately anxious	Moderate fidgety and restless	Moderate when hands are extended
5			
6			
7	Acute panic state/delirium	Severely agitated	Severe when hands are extended
Score	**Auditory Disturbance**	**Visual Disturbance**	**Tactile Disturbance**
0	Not present	Not present	Not present
1	Very mild harshness	Very mild photosensitivity	Very mild paresthesia
2	Mild harshness	Moderate photosensitivity	Mild paresthesia
3	Moderate harshness	Moderately severe photosensitivity	Moderate paresthesia
4	Moderately severe hallucinations	Moderately severe hallucinations	Moderately severe paresthesia

(continued)

TABLE 13–6 (Continued)		
5	Severe hallucinations	Severe hallucinations	Severe hallucinations
6	Extremely severe hallucinations	Extremely severe hallucinations	Extremely severe hallucinations
7	Continuous hallucinations	Continuous hallucinations	Continuous hallucinations
Score	**Orientation and Clouding of Sensorium**		
0	Oriented and can do serial additions		
1	Cannot do serial additions		
2	Disoriented to date by ≤ 2 days		
3	Disoriented to date by > 2 days		
4	Disoriented to place and or person		

Reproduced with permission: Sullivan, JT, Skyora K, Schneiderman J, et al. Assessment for alcohol scale (CIWA-Ar). *Br J Addict* 1987; 84:1353–1357

TABLE 13–6 (Continued)

ICU Admission Criteria

- Age > 40
- Cardiac disease (CHF, arrhythmia, angina, recent MI)
- Hemodynamic instability
- Acid–base disturbance
- Electrolyte disturbance
- Respiratory insufficiency
- Infection (severe)
- GI condition (pancreatitis, bleed, peritonitis, hepatic insufficiency)
- Persistent temp of >39°C (103°F)
- Rhabdomyolysis
- Renal insufficiency
- High dose of sedation requirement

TABLE 13–7: Alcohol Withdrawal Management

1. Thiamine 100 mg IV (prior to giving any glucose containing solution)

2. Folic acid 1 mg PO/IV PO daily

3. Multi vitamin 1 tab PO daily

4. Electrolytes: correct K^+, Mg, PO_4, and glucose

5. Psychomotor agitation: lorazepam (IV), diazepam (IV), chlordiazepoxide (PO), or oxazepam (PO)

Note: Lorazepam is minimally metabolized in liver (useful in patient with advanced cirrhosis).
  - Patients who are refractory to high-dose benzodiazepines, add phenobarbital or propofol.
  - Phenothiazines, butyrophenones, and Haldol should be avoided because they ↓ seizure threshold.

6. Seizure: benzodiazepines (lorazepam [IV], diazepam [IV])

Status epilepticus: benzodiazepines and consider phenytoin

  - Note: Carbamazepine should be avoided.

7. Tachycardia: β-blockers, such as propranolol (Inderal) and atenolol (Tenormin)

Medication dosing

  - Lorazepam 1–2 mg PO/IV q5-10min

  - Diazepam 5–20 mg PO/IV q5-10min

  - Phenobarbital 130–260 mg IV q15-20min

  - Propofol 1 mg/kg IV bolus then titrate infusion for sedation

TABLE 13–8: Aspirin (Salicylate) Overdose	
Signs and Symptoms	
• Nausea and vomiting	• Dehydration
• Altered mental status	• Tachypnea and hyperventilation
• Agitation	• Noncardiogenic pulmonary edema
• Tinnitus	• Hyperthermia
• Initially respiratory alkalosis then high anion gap metabolic acidosis	
Management	
• Supportive care	
• O_2	
• Volume resuscitate (be cautious in cerebral or pulmonary edema)	
• Activated charcoal (1 g/kg max up to 50 g PO)	
• Administer glucose in altered mental status even if concentration is normal	

(continued)

TABLE 13–8 (Continued)

- Alkalinize urine with sodium bicarbonate

  a. Give bolus of $NaHCO_3$ 2–3 meq/kg IV push (adult dosing)

  b. Then give maintenance of 132 meq $NaHCO_3$ in 1 $LD_5W \rightarrow$ at 250 mL/h (adult dose)

  c. For pediatric patient, use 100 meq $NaHCO_3$ in 1 L $D_5W \rightarrow$ at 1.5 to 2 times maintenance

Note: Do not use acetazolamide to alkalinize the urine.

- Monitor and correct electrolyte abnormalities and dehydration

- Consider hemodialysis in following conditions:

  1. Profoundly altered mental status

  2. Pulmonary or cerebral edema

  3. Renal failure

  4. Salicylate level > 100 mg/dL (7.2 mmol/L)

  5. Seizure

  6. Severe acidosis

  7. Fluid overload that prevents the administration of sodium bicarbonate

  8. Clinical deterioration despite aggressive and appropriate supportive care

TABLE 13–9: Benzodiazepine Poisoning

Signs and Symptoms

• Blurred vision	• Irritability
• Confusion	• Lethargy $\rightarrow$ coma
• Dizziness	• Poor muscle tone
• Hallucinations	• Respiratory depression
• Hypothermia	• Slurred speech

Management

• Flumazenil 0.2 mg IV over 30 s

    $\rightarrow$ 30 s later $\rightarrow$ 0.3 mg IV over 30 s

    $\rightarrow$ 30 s later $\rightarrow$ 0.5 mg (max: 5 mg)

• Avoid using flumazenil in chronic benzodiazepine users and mixed overdose $\rightarrow$ because it may cause seizure

Signs and Symptoms for Benzodiazepine Withdrawal

• Psychomotor agitation, combative	• Delirium
• Autonomic instability	• Seizure
• High BP	• Tachycardia

TABLE 13–10: Carbon Monoxide Poisoning

Signs and Symptoms

• Nausea	• Lethargy → coma
• Vomiting	• Malaise
• Headache	• Seizure

Management

- Give 100% O_2

- Obtain carboxyhemoglobin level

- Continue 100% O_2 until carboxyhemoglobin level is <5–10%

- Consider hyperbaric O_2 if unconscious, cardiac dysfunction, acidosis, neurologic focus, or pregnancy

TABLE 13–11: Cocaine Overdose

Signs and Symptoms

• Hypertension	• MI, stroke
• CNS bleed	• Bowel infarction
• Tachycardia	• Rhabdomyolysis
• Hyperpyrexia	• Diaphoresis
• Seizures	• Euphoria
• Arrhythmia (VT, V-fib)	• Obstetrical complication

Management

• Seizure: benzodiazepines

• Sedation: benzodiazepines

• Hyperthermia: water and fans (avoid phenothiazines)

• MI: see Chap. 2 (avoid β-blocker)

• Hypertension: clonidine, labetalol, nitroprusside, phentolamine, hydralazine (use during pregnancy) or Ca^+ channel blocker

• Tachyarrhythmia's: Ca^+ channel blocker and lidocaine (avoid β-blocker)

• Withdrawal: clonidine

• Rhabdomyolysis: fluids and urine alkalinization

Signs and Symptoms: Cocaine Withdrawal

• Dysphoria	• Lack of energy (fatigue)
• ↑Appetite	• Intense craving for the drug
• Hypersomnia—vivid dreams	• Dysphoric mood

TABLE 13–12: Digoxin Overdose

Signs and Symptoms

• Arrhythmia	• Color perception disturbance
• Abdominal pain	• Headache
• Blurred vision	• ↑ K$^+$
• Confusion/delirium	• Nausea/vomiting

Management

- Cardiac monitoring

- If serum K$^+$ > 5.5 meq/L → glucose + insulin, bicarbonate, Kayexalate (avoid calcium)

- Digibind (digoxin-specific antibody Fab fragments) indications:

  → Ventricular arrhythmias

  → Bradyarrhythmias unresponsive to atropine or pacemaker

  → Ingestion of >10 mg of digoxin in adults or ≥4 mg in children.

  → Plasma digoxin concentration above 10 ng/mL (13 mmol/L)

  → Serum K$^+$ > 5.5 meq/L in addition to life-threatening arrhythmia

TABLE 13–12 (Continued)

Administration of Digoxin-specific Fab Antibody Fragments (DSAF)

1. The IV dose is given over 15–30 min but can be given bolus in cardiac arrest

2. Dosing depends on steady state serum digitalis concentration or total amount ingested is known

3. If total amount ingested is known then follow:

   A. Total body load (TBL) = dose ingested (mg) for digitoxin (which has 100% bioavailability)

   B. Total body (TBL) = dose ingested (mg) × 0.8 for digoxin (which has 80% bioavailability)

   C. Number of vials = TBL/0.6

4. If steady state serum digitalis concentration (SDC) is not known

   A. Give 10 vials; repeat with another 10 vials if indicated

   B. Chronic toxicity: give 6 vials to an adult, one vial to a child

5. If the steady state serum digitalis concentration (SDC) is known

   A. TBL = (SDC [mg] × 5.6 × weight [kg])/1000

   B. TBL = (SDC [mg] × 0.56 × wt [kg])/1000

(Digitoxin has a much smaller volume of distribution is ≈ 0.56 L/kg)

   C. Calculation of the equimolar dose of DSAF

DSAF: its molecular weight (50,000) and that of digitoxin (781)

(continued)

TABLE 13–12 (Continued)

I. Dose of DSAF (mg) = TBL $\times$ (50,000/781) = TBL $\times$ 64
II. 1 vial of DSAF contains 40 mg, which neutralizes $\approx$ 0.6 mg of digoxin (0.6 $\times$ 64 = 40). Thus, number of vials = TBL/0.6
6. If we substitute this in equations A and B, where 0.6 divides roughly easily into the volumes of distribution for digoxin and digitoxin (5.6 and 0.56, respectively):
D. Number of vials for digoxin = (SDC $\times$ wt [kg])/100
E. Number of vials for digitoxin = (SDC $\times$ wt [kg]/1000
7. Hemodialysis or hemoperfusion can help control hyperkalemia or volume overload

Source with permission: Antman EM, Wenger TL, Butler VP, et al. Treatment of 150 cases of life-threatening digitalis intoxication with digoxin-specific Fab antibody fragments. Final report of a multicenter study. *Circulation.* 1990;81:1744.

TABLE 13–13: Ethylene Glycol Overdose

Signs and Symptoms

• Lethargy → coma	• Flank pain
• Tachypnea	• Renal failure (ATN)
• Pulmonary edema	• Calcium oxalate crystals in urine

Management

• Ethanol

• Sodium bicarbonate

• Dialysis: severe acidosis or renal failure

Note: Continue ethanol during dialysis.

• Thiamine

• Pyridoxine (B_6)

• Charcoal is not effective

TABLE 13–14: Methanol Intoxication

Signs and Symptoms

• Lethargy → coma	• CNS bleeding
• Blindness	• Pancreatitis

Management

• Ethanol

• Sodium bicarbonate

• Dialysis: severe acidosis or renal failure

Note: Continue ethanol during dialysis.

• Charcoal is not effective

TABLE 13–15: Opioid Intoxication (Heroin, Morphine, Meperidine, Fentanyl)

Signs and Symptoms

• Abnormal mental status	• Hypotension and bradycardia
• Miosis (pupillary constriction)	• Respiratory depression
• Pulmonary edema	• Acute respiratory acidosis
• Anaphylaxis	• Aspiration pneumonitis
• Coma	

Management

• Naloxone (Narcan) 0.4–0.8 mg IV (preferred), IM, intratracheal, Sub Q q2-3min as needed; may need to repeat doses q20min

(continued)

TABLE 13–15 (Continued)
Note
• If no response is observed after 10 mg, question the diagnosis.
• Use 0.1–0.2 mg increments in patients who are opioid dependent and in postoperative patients to avoid large cardiovascular changes.
• Duration of action of naloxone is 1–2 h
• Nalmefene: single Sub Q or IM dose of 1 mg may be effective in 5–15 min.
• IV: green-labeled product (1000 µg/mL); initial: 0.5 mg/70 kg
• May repeat with 1 mg/70 kg in 2–5 min.
• If opioid dependency is suspected, administer a challenge dose of 0.1 mg/70 kg
• For postoperative opioid depression: blue-labeled product (100 µg/mL); initial dose for non-opioid-dependent patient: 0.25 µg/kg followed by 0.25 µg/kg incremental doses at 2–5 min intervals.

TABLE 13–16: Opioid Withdrawal (Heroin, Morphine, Meperidine, Fentanyl)

Signs and Symptoms

• Mydriasis (pupillary dilatation)	• Lacrimation, rhinorrhea
• Piloerection	• Anorexia
• Yawning	• Nausea, vomiting, and diarrhea
• Sneezing	• Anxiety

Management

- Methadone: (see below table to calculate dosing), avoid in severe liver dz.

- Buprenorphine: 0.1–0.4 mg IM, slow IV q6h

- Clonidine: 1.2 mg/day in divided doses

(continued)

TABLE 13–16 (Continued)					
Methadone Dosing Table					
Signs and Symptoms	**0 H**	**6 H**	**12 H**	**18 H**	**24 H**
Mydriasis					
Rhinorrhea					
Lacrimation					
Goose flesh					
Nausea and vomiting					
Diarrhea					
Yawning					
Cramps					
Restlessness					
Voiced complaints					
Abnormal vital signs					

- 0 if no symptoms present, 1 point if the symptom is present; and 2 points if the symptom is severe
- Give methadone 1 mg for each point

TABLE 13–17: Organophosphate Intoxication

Signs and Symptoms

• CNS depression	• Hypersecretion
• Cramps	• Lacrimation
• Weakness	• Salivation
• Muscle fasciculation	• Sweating
• Diarrhea	• Miosis
• Abdominal cramps	• Urinary incontinence

Management

• Atropine 2–4 mg IV q15min until secretions stop (may require >1 g)

• Pralidoxime 1–2 g IV

• Decontaminate GI tract and skin

• Airway management is essential

TABLE 13–18: Tricyclic Antidepressants Overdose

Signs and Symptoms

• Coma	• Hypotension
• Respiratory depression	• Arrhythmia
• Seizure	• Cardiac conduction defect

ECG Changes

• Sinus tachycardia, VT, PVCs	• Prolonged QT → torsades de pointes
• QRS > 100 ms	• ↑ PR interval

Management

- Lavage
- Activated charcoal
- Monitor acid–base: keep pH at 7.5
- If hypotension: IVF and pressors
- If seizure: benzodiazepines
- If conduction block: consider pacer
- If VT or PVCs: consider lidocaine or magnesium
- Indication for sodium bicarbonate
  1. Hypotension
  2. Arrhythmia
  3. Hemodynamic stable patient with QRS > 100 ms
  4. Seizures

TABLE 13-19: Toxins and Antidotes

Toxin	Antidotes	Toxin	Antidotes
Acetaminophen	*N*-Acetylcysteine	Ethylene glycol	Ethanol
Alcohol	Naloxone	Heparin	Protamine sulfate
Anticholinergic	Physostigmine	Iron	Deferoxamine
β-Blocker	Glucagon	Isoniazid	Pyridoxine
Benzodiazepines	Flumazenil	Methanol	Ethanol
Ca$^+$ channel blocker	Calcium	Narcotics	Naloxone
Carbon monoxide	100% O_2, hyperbaric O_2	Nitrates	Methylene blue
Cyanide	Sodium nitrate	Organophosphate	Atropine, pralidoxime
	Sodium thiosulfate	Phenothiazines	Benadryl
Digitalis	Digoxin FAB	Warfarin	Vitamin K

14
Neonatology

TABLE 14–1: Note

- Infant screening Web site: www.NeoGenScreening.com

- Preterm infant: <36 weeks, should get car seat test prior to discharge

- SGA: <2500 g, should be placed in incubator, check glucose level

- LGA: >4000 g

- SGA and preterm babies should start feeding in 1–2 h of conception

- Macrosomia: >4500 g infant from diabetic mother or >5000 g infant from nondiabetic mother

- Infant's weight should be checked at 24 h

- Transcutaneous bilirubin check at 36 h

- If the baby is jaundiced and mother with Rh(−) blood type → check baby's blood type and comb

- Teen pregnancy: order social work consult

- Infant should void and have BM within 24–48 h

- Infant should lose up to 10% of body weight from birth in first 5–7 days

- Consider giving hepatitis B vaccine immunization prior to discharge

- Mother with C-section usually stays in hospital for up to 72 h

- If mother is GBS (+) → baby should be observed for up to 48 h for signs of infection

- ♀: may have bloody vaginal discharge for first few days

- ♂: do not perform circumcision until infant voids

TABLE 14–2: Check for Following Status in Mother

• Blood type	• RPR
• Antibody	• HIV (optional)
• Hep Bs Ag	• HSV (optional)
• GBS	• Tox. screen (optional)
• Rubella	

A. GBS (+) Status in Mother

• If mother is GBS (+) → observe infant for at least 72 h for following:

1. Sepsis

2. Pneumonia

3. Respiratory distress

4. Leukopenia

5. Meningitis

B. Hepatitis B Vaccination in Infant

• If mother is Hep Bs Ag (−) → give Hep B vaccine in 24–72 h

• If mother is Hep Bs Ag (+) → give Hep B vaccine in 72 h + give HBIG in 12 h

• If hepatitis status unknown → give Hep B vaccine in 24–72 h and √ hepatitis status of mother

(continued)

TABLE 14–2 (Continued)
C. Rubella Nonimmune Status in Mother
• If mother is not rubella immune vaccinate mother with rubella vaccine postpartum
D. Positive Syphilis Serology in Mother and Infant
• If mother is RPR+ → check infant for FTA-ABS IgM and IgG
• If infant has FTA-ABS IgM → rule out CNS infection

TABLE 14–3: Physical Examination

1. Gen: check skin for color (jaundice)

2. HEENT: check for caput succedaneum/cephalhematoma and palpate sutures

   - Check for red reflex (absent in patient with retinoblastoma or cataract)

   - Check for conjunctival hemorrhage

   - Check for low set ears (low set ears represents Down's syndrome)

   - Check the hard palate and soft palate (make sure it's intact)

3. Neck: check for any remnant openings in the neck

4. Chest: check clavicle for crepitation (represents fracture)

   - Check the lungs

5. CVS: check for heart murmur

6. Abd: check for abdominal mass

7. Ext: count all fingers and toes, check tone

   - Check palmar crease (single palmar crease may represents Down's syndrome [normal in 5%])

   - Check for femoral pulses

8. Genitals: male: check for descended testes, hypospadias or epispadias

9. Hip: check for any clicks or clunks during hip examination

(continued)

TABLE 14–3 (Continued)

10. Back: check the back for any openings or dimpling

   • Check for skin tags or tuft of hair (ear, back)

11. Reflexes: suck reflex, plantar reflex, Moro reflex, startle reflex, and grasp reflex

Document Following in the Chart

• Birth weight	• Length
• Head circumference	• Temperature
• Bottle vs. breast feeding	• Voiding
• Ask mother (circumcision vs. noncircumcision)	• Stooling
• Do not perform circumcision until ♂ infant voids	• APGAR scores
• Transcutaneous bilirubin (TCB) at 36 h	• Tox. screen, if high-risk infant

Consults and Tests Prior to Discharge

• Lactation	• Hearing
• Social work	• Car seat test
• Home health	

TABLE 14–4: Take-home Instructions

- **Feeding (Breast feeding vs. bottle feeding)**

  1. Breast feeding babies should be fed 8–12 times a day in first week

  2. Infant should be burped frequently

  3. Do not give plain or sugar water

  4. Do not give whole milk the first year of life

  5. Do not give solid foods or drinks except for breast milk or formula

- **Bathing**

  1. Infant should receive sponge bath until cord falls off

  2. Can use lukewarm water or may use mild soap shampoo

  3. There is no need to use oils, creams, lotions, or powders

  4. Do not use Q-tips to clean infant's ears or nose

- **Cord care**

  1. Area surrounding cord should be kept dry and clean

  2. Clean base of the cord with alcohol about 3–4 times per day with Q-tip

  3. Cord usually falls off around 10–14 days

  4. Contact your pediatrician if cord area becomes red and inflamed and is oozing

- **Genital care (circumcised vs. uncircumcised)**

  1. If male infant is circumcised, apply Vaseline to the tip of the penis to prevent it from sticking to diaper

(continued)

TABLE 14–4 (Continued)

2. Circumcision usually heals within 1 week

3. If circumcised male has unusual bleeding, swelling, or rash over the circumcised area, call pediatrician

4. Infant with uncircumcised penis should have daily washing with gentle soap and water

5. There is no need to retract the foreskin in uncircumcised penis for cleaning

- **Stooling**

  1. Infant may have bowel movement (BM) after each feeding but it's normal to have one every other day

  2. Call your pediatrician if stool is hard, green in color, or watery

- **Clothing**

  1. Dress the baby according to the outside temperature (do not under dress or over dress)

- **Environment**

  1. Avoid crowded places

  2. Avoid contact with individuals who are sick

- **Contact PCP if:**

  1. If temp (rectal) > 100.4°F (>38°C) or axillary > 99.5°F (>37.6°C)

  2. Decrease in activity (sleeps all the time and hard to awaken)

  3. Infant is unusually irritable

  4. Infant has difficulty breathing

  5. Infant has unusual rash

TABLE 14–5: Jaundice in Neonate

Total Cutaneous Bilirubin (TCB) ≈ Total Serum Bilirubin (TSB)

Physiologic	Pathologic
• Starts > 24 h	• Starts < 24 h
• Disappears in 1 week	• Lasts >1 week
• Total bilirubin: <17	• Total bilirubin: >17
• Direct bilirubin: <2	• Direct bilirubin: >2
Etiology	
• Underdeveloped liver	• ↑ Hemolysis (Rh and ABO incompatibility)
• ↑ Enterohepatic reabsorption	• Crigler-Najar syndrome
	• Dubin-Johnson syndrome
	• Duodenal atresia
	• Intestinal obstruction
	• Annular pancreas
Complication	
• Kernicterus: deposition of unconjugated bilirubin in basal ganglia	
It can cause cerebral palsy, hearing loss, vision and teeth problems and sometimes can cause mental retardation	

(continued)

TABLE 14–5 (Continued)					
Labs: Infant with Jaundice that Occurs < 24 H					
• Bilirubin total		• Hemoglobin and hematocrit			
• Bilirubin direct		• Blood type			
• Reticulocyte count		• Coombs (direct/indirect)			
Treatment of High Bilirubin for Preterm Infant					
Birth weight	<1250 g	<1500 g	<2000 g	<2500 g	>2500 g
Uncomplicated	>13 mg/dL	>15 mg/dL	>17 mg/dL	>18 mg/dL	>20 mg/dL
Complicated	>10 mg/dL	>13 mg/dL	>15 mg/dL	>17 mg/dL	>18 mg/dL
Treatment of High bilirubin for Term Infant					
	25–48 h of age	49–72 h of age		>73 h of age	
Uncomplicated	15–25 mg/dL	18–30 mg/dL		20–30 mg/dL	
Complicated	12 mg/dL or higher	15 mg/dL or higher		17 mg/dL or higher	

TABLE 14–5 (Continued)

Note

- If bilirubin ≥ 25 mg/dL at 25–48 h of age consider exchange transfusion.

- If bilirubin ≥ 30 mg/dL at ≥49 h consider exchange transfusion.

Treatment Modalities for Neonate with Jaundice and High Bilirubin

- Phototherapy (single, double)

- Bili-Blanket

- IVF

- Exchange transfusion

15
OB/GYN

TABLE 15–1: Abbreviations

G P T P A L

G = Gravid (number of pregnancies)
P = Para (number of deliveries to age of viability, which is >23 weeks)
T = Full Term deliveries
P = Preterm deliveries
A = Abortions
L = Currently living children

TABLE 15–2: OB Visit Schedule

- Estimated date of confinement (EDC) = 1st day of LMP + 7 days + 9 months

- Offer prenatal vitamins with iron + folic acid on 1st OB visit

- Preterm < 37, postterm > 42

1st OB Visit Lab	16–20 Weeks	32 Weeks
Hb/HCT	• Triple screen test 1. β-HCG 2. AFP 3. Estradiol • PAPP at 15 week optional • Ultrasound: for gestational age	Repeat 1 h 50 g glucola if previous 1 h glucola >140 and 3 h was WNL
Blood type and Rh		
Antibody screen		
RPR/VDRL		
Rubella Ab		**32–36 Weeks**
Hep Bs Ag		US (fetal survey)—prn
UA, urine C&S		
Pap (thin prep)	**24–28 Weeks**	**35–37 Weeks**
Wet prep	1 h 50 g glucola → if >140 then → check 3 h OGTT[b]	Gonorrhea Cx[a]
Gonorrhea Cx[a]		Chlamydia Cx[a]

TABLE 15–2 (Continued)		
Chlamydia Cx[a]	CBC (H&H)	Group B Strep Cx (GBS)
PPD	**28 Weeks**	**>40 Weeks**
HIV screen	If Rh(−) → give RhoGAM[c]	NST
TSH screen		**41 Weeks**
Sickle cell screen (hemoglobin electrophoresis)		BPP
Tay-Sachs dz. Screen		**Postpartum**
Cystic fibrosis		H&H at 12–18 h
VZV titer: if patient has no history of exposure		RhoGAM[d]
Genetic screening if >35 years		
Urine Tox. screen[a]		
Visit Schedule		**Every Visit**
<28 Weeks → q4wk		Problems and concerns
28 and 36 Weeks → q2-4wk		Fetal well-being (fetal movement)
>36 Weeks– 40→q1-2wk		Assess fetal heart tone
>40 Weeks → q3-7day		Assess fundal height
		Signs of toxemia (BP and protein in UA)
Abbreviation: PAPP, pregnancy associated plasma protein.		

(continued)

TABLE 15–2 (Continued)
Note
• PAPP detects Down's syndrome in 1st trimester, if (+) → consider chorionic villous sampling.
• If patient has high AFP → order US to confirm gestational age and R/O twin, or fetal demise.
• Nitrazine test → positive (blue) → detects amniotic fluid
→ False positive Nitrazine test: semen/blood/bacterial vaginosis
• If Group B Strep (+) management (see Table 15–16)
• If urine culture grows Group B Strep > 100k CFU → give amoxicillin 500 mg bid × 7–10 days.
And there is no need to check for Group B Strep at 36 weeks but treat patient during labor with Abx.
• Mother → Hep Bs Ag (−) → give mother Hep B vaccine within 12 h.
→ Hep Bs Ag (+) → give Hep B vaccine within 24–72 h and immunoglobulin in 12 h.
→ Hep B status unknown → give Hep B vaccine within 12 h, send for Hep B serology.

[a]Perform in high-risk patient.
[b]3 h Glucola test: normal values (2/4); Fasting < 105; 1 h < 190; 2 h < 165; 3 h < 145.
[c]Perform Rh antibody screen prior to administration, if (−) then administer RhoGAM 300 µg IM.
[d]RhoGAM should be given postpartum if mother is Rh (−) and baby is Rh (+). Weight gain in pregnancy should be approximate 20–35 lb.

TABLE 15–3: Pregnancy Landmarks

12 Weeks	Uterus at symphysis pubis, able to hear fetal heart tone with Doppler
16 Weeks	Uterus at midpoint between symphysis pubis and umbilicus
20 Weeks	Uterus at umbilicus
20–37 Weeks	Uterus should measure according to the weeks of gestation in cm

TABLE 15–4: Preterm Labor (PTL)

ACOG Defines as

- Regular contractions (see below) with cervical change before 37 weeks' gestation

- Four regular contractions in 20 min

- Eight regular contractions in 60 min with PROM → progressive cervical change

  → Effacement > 80%

  → Cervical dilation > 1 cm

Maternal Risk Factors

Age (<18 and >40)	Prior preterm birth
Race (nonwhite)	Prior 2nd trimester abortion
Poverty	Psychological stress
Smoking	Poor nutrition
Drugs/ETOH	Low prepregnancy weight and gain

Preterm Labor (PTL) Index (with Membrane Intact)

Scores	0	1	2	3	4
Uterine contraction	None	<6/h	≥6/h	–	–
Bleeding (gram)	None	<10/h	≥10/ h	–	–
Cervical dilatation (cm)	None	1 to <2	2–3	3 to <4	≥4

- If score is > 3 there is high risk of preterm delivery

TABLE 15–4 (Continued)

Other risk factors

- Anatomic anomaly: fibroids, placenta previa

- Increased volume: multiple gestation, polyhydramnios

- Trauma/abruption

- Cervical incompetence

- Infection

Consider the following testing modalities

Consider ultrasound to determine cervical length

Biochemical markers

• Fetal fibronectin (swab sample of vaginal secretion)	
• IL-6	• Salivary estriol
• Progesterone	• Estradiol-17B

TABLE 15–5: Tocolysis

- Nifedipine 5–10 mg PO/SL q15-20min (max: 30–40 mg) then 10–20 mg q3-8h or

  - Avoid if: magnesium sulfate is at 1 g/h

  - Monitor for hypotension and reflex tachycardia

- Magnesium sulfate 4–6 g IV over 10–20 min then 1 g/h IV drip or

  - Check Mg level 1 h after starting Mg and then every 4 h

  - Check DTR (reflexes)

  - Monitor respiration and urine output

  - Decrease or hold if: absent DTR, RR < 10, urine output < 25–40 mL/h

  - Mg toxicity: hold and give calcium gluconate 10% solution 10 mL IV over 10 min

- Terbutaline 0.25 mg Sub Q q1-4h or 2.5–10 mg PO q4-6h

  - Or give 0.005 mg /min IV and ↑ by 0.05 mg/min q10min (max: 0.08 mg/min)

  - Or Sub Q pump basal rate 0.05–0.1 mg/h

- Ritodrine 0.05 mg/min IV ↑ by 0.05 mg/min q10min (max: 0.35 mg/min) or

  - Hold if fetal heart rate: >180 or <100, maternal SBP < 90, RR > 28, heart rate > 120, chest pain

- Indomethacin consider OB consult prior to use due to its effect on IVH and PDA closure or

  - 50–100 mg rectal suppository then 25 mg PO qid for 24 h

  - 50 mg PO then 25 mg PO q4h for 24 h

  - 100 mg vaginal suppository q12h × 2 doses

TABLE 15–6: Stages of Labor	
1st Stage (Divided into 2 Phases)	**2nd Stage (Complete Cervical Dilation–Delivery of Baby)**
Nulliparity: <6–18 h	Nulliparous: <3 h; descent: >1 cm/h
Multiparity: <2–10 h	Multiparous: <1 h; descent: >2 cm/h
A. Latent phase (cervical dilation: 0–4 cm)	
Rx: Rest/morphine 15–20 mg or epidural	**3rd Stage (Birth of the Baby to the Delivery of Placenta)**
B. Active phase (4–10 cm)	Placenta delivery: <30 min
Nulliparity: >1.2 cm/h	Rx: Pitocin with delivery of anterior shoulder
Multiparity: >1.4 cm/h	(for active management of labor to reduce PPH)
Rx: Amniotomy and/or pitocin for ↑ labor/epidural and Stadol for analgesia	

TABLE 15–7: Postpartum Hemorrhage Management

- Assess patient and check vitals

- OB consult may be required if patient is unstable

Etiologies

Uterine atony	Laceration (cervical, vaginal)	
Retain tissue	Bleeding diathesis	

Risk of atony is increased with

Uterine over distention	Multiparity	Preeclampsia
Chorioamnionitis	General anesthesia	Magnesium sulfate

1. Uterine massage

2. Consider type, cross, and transfuse PRBC

3. Birth canal inspection and then manual uterine inspection

4. Uterine gauze packing

5. Oxytocin 10–20 units IM or IV 40–80 units in 1 L of NS → at 200–250 mL/h

6. Methylergonovine 0.2 mg IM and/or 0.2 mg PO q2-8h (avoid in patient with ↑ BP or CAD)

7. Carboprost 0.25–1 mg IM or intramyometrium q15min (max: 2 mg) (avoid in asthma, renal, hepatic, or cardiac disease)

8. Misoprostol 800–1000 µg per rectum

9. Hysterectomy

TABLE 15–8: Postcoital Contraception

- Levonorgestrel (Plan B 0.75 mg 1 tab PO × 1 now and 0.75 mg 1 tab PO × 1 in 12 h (2 doses of 0.75 mg can be taken at the same time but its been associated with nausea)

- Preven 2 tab (ethinyl estradiol 100 μg + levonorgestrel 0.75 mg) now and 2 tab in 12 h

- Lo/Ovral 4 tab (ethinyl estradiol 120 μg + levonorgestrel 0.60 mg) now and 2 tab in 12 h

- Ovral 2 tab (ethinyl estradiol 100 μg + levonorgestrel 0.50 mg) now and 2 tab in 12 h

TABLE 15–9: Indication for RhoGAM

If mother is Rh (−) → give RhoGAM at 28 weeks and if newborn is Rh (+) → also give RhoGAM within 72 h postpartum (give RhoGAM after the following procedures)

- After amniocentesis

- After D and C

- After abortion

- RhoGAM dosage is 300 μg IM (Perform Rh antibody screen prior to administration, administer only if antibody screen is negative)

TABLE 15–10: Premature Rupture of Membrane (PROM)

Condition	Labs
Pooling of fluid seen during speculum examination	CBC with diff
Nitrazine test → detects amniotic fluid positive (blue)	GBS Cx
Ferning → Christmas tree pattern (under microscopy)	Ultrasound
Fetal fibronectin (swab vaginal secretion)	Amniocentesis

PROM management

Assess fetal well-being: fetal size, presentation, and fetal heart rate

Hydration

Bed rest

Biophysical profile				
Scoring	2	+ NST	2	Fetal movement
	2	Fetal tone	2	Respiration
	2	Amniotic fluid		
1. If total score is <8 or		• Consider delivery, repeat BPP within 24 h, or perinatology consult		
2. If amniotic fluid is 0 or				
3. If poor NST				

TABLE 15–10 (Continued)

Amniotic fluid Index

- Divide uterus into four quadrants (Use linea nigra for right and left divisions and umbilicus for upper and lower quadrants)

- Measure maximum width (in centimeter) of each quadrant that is not containing cord/fetal extremity

- Normal—5.1–25 cm

- Oligohydramnios—0–5 cm

- Polyhydramnios—>25 cm

TABLE 15–11: Tests, Scores, and Monitoring

Bishop Scoring

Description	Scoring			
	0	**1**	**2**	**3**
Dilatation (cm)	0	1–2	3–4	5–6
Effacement	0–30%	40–50%	60–70%	>80%
Station	−3	−2	−1 to 0	+1 to +2
Consistency	Firm	Medium	Soft	
Position	Posterior	Mid	Anterior	

- If score is >7 → cervix is favorable for spontaneous labor or induced labor

Nonstress testing

- Fetal stimulation can be performed manually, acoustically, or administration of glucose beverage

Reactive	• 2 accelerations in 20 min of fetal heart rate, 15 bpm above baseline lasting 15 s
Nonreactive	• Absence of 2 accelerations in 20 min

Contraction Stress Testing

Positive	• Persistent late or significant variable deceleration after >50% of contraction without uterine hyperstimulation
Negative	• No late or significant variable deceleration with contractions of at least 3 in 10 min

TABLE 15–11 (Continued)

Electronic Fetal Monitoring (EFM)

- Bradycardia → mild: 100–120 (common with postdates)

  → Moderate: 80–100

  → Severe: < 80 lasting for > 3 min (severe hypoxia)

- Tachycardia → mild: 160–180

  → Moderate: 180–200 (fever)

  → Severe: >200 (tachyarrhythmia)

- Variability: constant variation of heart rate; correlates with good outcome

  → Decreased variability: 2° → baby sleeping, medication

  (Analgesics, anesthetics, Mg)

  → Increased (>25 bpm): 2° → hypoxia or cord compression

- Accelerations: ↑ heart rate of 15 bpm lasting > 15 s (fetal well-being)

- Deceleration: → mild: >80 bpm for < 30 s

  → Moderate: 70–80 bpm for 30–60 s

  → Severe: <70 bpm for >60 s

- Early: 2° from head compression (reassuring)

- Late: → begin after peak of contraction and run after contraction (nonreassuring)

  → 2° Uteroplacental insufficiency → needs evaluation

- Variable: cord compression, decreased amniotic fluid

TABLE 15–12: Vaginal Bleeding in Pregnancy	
Early in Pregnancy	**Late in Pregnancy**
Miscarriage	Placenta previa
Ectopic pregnancy	Placenta abruptio
Trophoblastic disease	Vasa previa (rupture)
	Uterine scar disruption
Miscellaneous Etiologies in Early and Late Pregnancy	
Vaginal trauma	Cervical polyp
Cervical cancer	Cervicitis

TABLE 15–13: Ectopic Pregnancy

Signs and symptoms

- Amenorrhea

- Abnormal vaginal bleeding

- Abdominal pain

- Positive β-HCG in the absence of intrauterine pregnancy by ultrasound

- Note: The absence of an intrauterine gestational sac at β-HCG concentrations > 2000 IU/L strongly suggests an ectopic pregnancy

- Risk factors: Prior ectopic, Hx of PID, Hx of STDs, IUD use, and tubal ligation

- Evaluate fetal cardiac activity with TVUS (transvaginal ultrasound)

Management

- Methotrexate therapy (requires β-HCG monitoring for approximately 1 year)

- Laparotomy or laparoscopic surgical removal

  Indications for surgical removal:

  1. Ruptured ectopic, especially in hemodynamically unstable patient

  2. Inability to comply with posttreatment monitoring after medical Rx

- Expectant management

TABLE 15–14: Hyperemesis Gravidarum

- Persistent vomiting at all times of the day not just in the morning

- Differential: CBC, electrolytes, U/A, urine tox, LFT, pelvic U/S

- Management: 1. Hydration with IVF if dehydration noted

    2. Consider small frequent meals ($\uparrow$ complex carbohydrates)

    3. Pyridoxine (B_6) 25–50 mg

    4. Doxylamine 12.5–25 mg PO q6-8h

    5. Zofran 4 mg PO/IV q6h

TABLE 15–15: Preeclampsia

Mild Preeclampsia and Severe Eclampsia Classification

	BP	Proteinuria	Signs and Symptoms
Mild preeclampsia	>140/90 × 2 (6 h apart)	>+1 dipstick	>5 lb wt. gain in 1 week
	Or 30/15 ↑ over baseline	>300 mg/24 h	
Severe eclampsia	>160/110 × 2 (6 h apart)	>+2 dipstick × 2	Oliguria <500 mL/24 h
		4 h apart	Visual disturbance
		>3.5–5 g/24 h	Headache
			Pulmonary edema
			Epigastric/RUQ pain
			↑ LFTs

(continued)

TABLE 15–15 (Continued)

		Thrombocytopenia		
Eclampsia	>160/110 × 2 (6 h apart)	> +2 dipstick × 2	Seizure	
		4 h apart		
		>3.5–5 g/24 h		

Preeclampsia Labs

• CBC with platelets	• Spot urine protein:creatinine ratio (positive if >0.2)	• BUN/creatinine
• Liver function test	Or	• Uric acid
• LDH	• UA, 24 h urine protein (positive if >300 mg) and creatinine	• PT/PTT
• Bilirubin	• Consider urine tox. Screen	• Uric acid level

Severe Preeclampsia, HELLP Syndrome LAB (In Addition to Above Labs)		
• Peripheral smear	• Fibrinogen	• D-dimer
• If PTT is prolonged → order anticardiolipin antibodies and lupus anticoagulant		
Note		
• Spot urine protein:creatinine ratio: <2 or <300 mg/24 h is normal.		
• Severe eclampsia: repeat labs q4-6h.		
• Mild preeclampsia: repeat labs everyday.		
• If platelet is noted to be low: repeat platelets q4h during labor.		
• If patient is on Mg for treatment → check Mg levels (therapeutic level 5–8 mg/dL).		
→ Check serial DTRs.		
• Consider NST, BPP.		

(continued)

TABLE 15–15 (Continued)

Mild Preeclampsia Treatment

If term → hasten delivery

If preterm → bed rest and monitor for symptoms, NST, BPP

  → Consider magnesium sulfate

Severe Preeclampsia/Eclampsia Treatment

- NPO and O_2
- BP management: → hydralazine 2.5–10 mg IV q20min or

  → Labetalol 10–20 mg IV q10-20min or

  → Nifedipine 10–20 mg SL/PO q20min (caution: causes hypotension with $MgSO_4$)

  (Use nifedipine until diastolic [DBP] < 100 then maintain DBP = 100)

- Seizure prophylaxis:

  → Magnesium sulfate 4–6 g IV over 10–20 min then 1–4 g/h IV drip (continue postpartum 24–48 h)

→ Continue infusion for 24–48 h postpartum

→ Check Mg level 1 h after starting Mg and then every 4 h

→ Therapeutic level 5–8 mg/dL

→ Check DTR (reflexes), monitor respiration and urine output

→ Decrease or hold if : absent DTR, RR < 10, urine output < 25–40 mL/h

→ If Mg toxicity: hold and give calcium gluconate 10% solution 10 mL IV over 10 min

→ Continue up to 24 h postpartum

• Recurrent seizure: → in addition to prophylactic magnesium sulfate, give magnesium sulfate 2 g IV

→ Amobarbital 250 mg in 10 mL NS IV over 3–4 min

→ Diazepam 5–10 mg IV slow push

→ Pentobarbital 125 mg IV

• Consider corticosteroid if 24–34 weeks and consult OB

(continued)

TABLE 15–15 (Continued)

Magnesium level and clinical signs

Magnesium Level (mg/dL)	Clinical Signs
1.3–2.6	Normal
4–8	Therapeutic
8–10	Loss of patellar reflex
10–13	Somnolence
12–15	Respiratory depression
15–17	Paralysis
30–25	Cardiac arrest

Antidote: Calcium gluconate 1 g IV over 3 min.

TABLE 15–16: Group B Strep (GBS [+]) Management

- Penicillin G 5 million units IV then 2.5 million units IV q4h until delivery 1st line

- Ampicillin 2 g IV then 1 g IV q4h 2nd line

- If penicillin allergy: clindamycin 900 mg IV q8h or erythromycin 500 mg IV q6h

TABLE 15–17: Amenorrhea (1st and 2nd)

Primary amenorrhea evaluation

- 1° amenorrhea: no menses by age 16 years

- It is due to genetic or a congenital defect

- Evaluate breast development and other secondary characteristics

- Check FSH level

  - If ↑ FSH and no breast development → gonadal dysgenesis

  - If ↑ FSH is elevated → order karyotype (gonadal dysgenesis is associated with 46,XY)

- Evaluate presence or absence of cervix

- Order ultrasound to evaluate the presence or absence of uterus

  - If uterus is missing → Dx: Müllerian

TABLE 15-17 (Continued)

Secondary amenorrhea evaluation

- Absence of menses for more than three cycle intervals or six months in women who were previously menstruating

- Check: β-HCG, prolactin level, and TSH level

- If all above tests are normal then consider progestin challenge; progestin PO × 5–7 days or IM × 10 days

  → If bleeding occurs → means there is either hypothalamic dysfunction or premature ovarian failure

- To differentiate between hypothalamic dysfunction and premature ovarian failure, check FSH.

  - Low FSH: hypothalamic dysfunction

  - High FSH: ovarian failure

- Testosterone level

TABLE 15–18: Contraception Modalities

A. OCP combined (estrogen and progestin)

Effectiveness 0.3% (failure rate higher in teenagers)

- A pack consists of 21 pills plus may or may not contain 7 placebo pills, bleeding occurs q month

- Start on 1st day of the menses or 1st Sunday after menses begin

- Patient who is postpartum and breast feeding: if <6 months after delivery, wait until baby is receiving significant nutritional supplement

- Patient who is postpartum and not breast feeding: wait at least 3 weeks after delivery to abate hypercoagulable state

B. Patches—Ortho Evra weekly patch, effectiveness 0.3–0.6%

- A pack consists 3 patches, 1 patch is worn for 1 week, 4th week is patch free to permit bleeding.

- Applied to upper outer arm or to upper torso (except for the breast), Δ location q month.

- Place 1st patch on 1st day of menstrual period

- Injection is given within 1st 5 days of the start of menses

- Postpartum: 1st injection is given prior to hospital discharge, delay in severe obstetrical blood loss

- Do not massage area where shot was given.

- Return in 11–13 weeks for next injection (use abstinence after 13 weeks)

- Theoretically menstruation does not occur when on Depo-Provera

TABLE 15–19: Endometriosis Treatment

- Danazol 800 mg/day in divided doses

- OCP (continuous or cyclic)

- Medroxyprogesterone suspension 100 mg IM q2wks × 2 months → 200 mg IM × 4 months

- Medroxyprogesterone 5–20 mg PO/day

- Norethindrone acetate 5 mg/day × 2 weeks then ↑ by 2.5 mg/day every 2 weeks up to 15 mg/day

- Leuprolide 3.75 mg IM every month for 6 months

- Goserelin 3.6 mg Sub Q (in upper abdominal wall) every 28 days

- Nafarelin 400 mg per day: 1 spray in 1 nostril in a.m.; 1 spray in other nostril in p.m.; start treatment on day 2–4 of menstrual cycle

- Hysterectomy

- Oophorectomy

TABLE 15–20: Mastitis

- Warm compresses

- Dicloxacillin 500 mg PO q6h or

- Cefazolin 1 g IV q8h or

- Clindamycin 300 mg PO q6h or

- Vancomycin 1 g IV q12h

16
Pediatrics

TABLE 16–1: Normal Vital Signs

Age (Weight, kg)	Systolic BP (Min–Max)	Heart Rate (Min–Max)	Respiration Rate (Min–Max)
Preemie (1–2)	50–70	90–180	30–60
Newborn (3.5)	50–70	90–180	30–60
6 Months (7)	65–106	85–170	24–40
1 Year (10)	72–110	80–140	20–40
3 Years (15)	78–114	80–130	20–30
6 Years (20)	80–116	70–120	18–25
8 Years (25)	84–122	70–110	18–25
10 Years (30)	90–130	65–110	16–20
12 Years (40)	94–136	60–110	14–20
15 Years (50)	100–140	55–100	12–20
18 Years (65)	104–140	50–90	12–18

Pearls

- Weight in kg (for 1–8 years) = $10 + (2 \times$ patient's age in years)
- Least acceptable systolic BP: birth to 1 month = 60

  1 month to 1 year = 70

  >1 year = 70 + age in years
- Endotracheal tube size = (age in years/4) + 4

(continued)

TABLE 16–1 (Continued)			
APGAR Score			
Description	**Score**		
	0	1	2
Appearance (color)	Blue/pale	Blue	Pink
Pulse	Absent	<100	≥100
Grimace	None	Grimace	Good cry
Activity (tone)	Limp/floppy	Some flexion	Active (normal tone)
Respiratory rate	Absent	Slow irregular	Regular sustained

- Apgar score is monitored at birth and at 5 min
- APGAR at 5 min is >7 → infant does not require any assistance
- APGAR at 5 min is 4–6 →
  1. Re-dry the infant
  2. Continue stimulation by rubbing the feet, chest, and spine.
  3. Provide assistance with ventilation using 100 % O_2
  4. Monitor Heart rate, respiration, tone, and color

TABLE 16–2: Developmental Milestones

1 Month	2 Months
• Raises head from prone	• Lifts chest off table
• Tight grasp	• Visually follows objects past midline
• Alerts to sound	• Smiles
4 Months	**6 Months**
• Rolls over	• Sits unsupported
• Brings hands to mouth	• Babbles
• Laughs	• Recognizes strangers
• Follows moving objects	• Weight doubles from birth
9 Months	**12 Months**
• Crawls	• Walks alone without support
• Pulls to stand	• Pincer grasp
• Throws objects	• Uses two words besides "mama, dada"
• Says "mama, dada", stranger anxiety	• Start baby on whole milk and discontinue bottle feeding
• Waves "bye bye"	• Weight triples from birth

(continued)

TABLE 16–2 (Continued)	
15 Months	**18 Months**
• Creeps up stairs	• Runs
• Scribbles	• Throws objects from standing
• Plays ball	• Scribbles spontaneously
• Follows one step command	• Has 7–10-word vocabulary
• Uses 4–6 words	• Knows 5 body parts
• Uses cup and spoon	• Copies parents in chores (i.e., cleaning)
24 Months	**3 Years**
• Walks up and down steps without help	• Pedals tricycles
• Strokes with pen or pencil	• Copies a circle
• Uses 2-word sentences	• Washes and dries hands
• Uses 2-step commands	• Uses 3-word sentences
	• Uses plurals

TABLE 16–2 (Continued)	
4 Years	**5 Years**
• Hops, skips	• Jumps over low obstacles
• Dresses self	• Ties shoes
• Buttons clothing	• Speech: completely understandable
• Knows colors	• Prints first name
• Plays with children in a group	• Helps with household tasks

Counseling parents about:
   A. Using car seat
   B. Working fire alarm in the house
   C. Bike helmet

TABLE 16–3: Tanner Staging

Tanner Staging for Female

Stage	I	II	III	IV	V
Breast	No budding	Budding	Small breast	Areola and papilla form	Adult size breast
Pubic hair	No hair	Growth of slightly pigmented hair	Dark, coarse, beginning to curl	Adult characteristics but not adult distribution	Adult pubic hair

Tanner Staging for Male

Stage	I	II	III	IV	V
Testes	No testicular enlargement	Testicular enlargement	↑ length of penis	Further penile enlargement, darkening of scrotal skin	Adult size penis
Pubic hair	No hair	Growth of slightly pigmented hair	Dark, coarse, beginning to curl	Adult characteristics but not adult distribution	Adult pubic hair

TABLE 16–4: Pediatric Immunization Schedule					
Birth	Hep B #1				
2 Months	Hep B #2	DTaP #1	Hib #1	IPV #1	PCV#1
4 Months		DTaP #2	Hib #2	IPV #2	PCV#2
6 Months	Hep B #3	DTaP #3	Hib #3	IPV #3	PCV#3
6 Months	Influenza (yearly)				
12–15 Months	MMR #1		Hib #4		PCV#4
12–18 Months	Varicella[a]				
12 Months	Hepatitis A				
15–18 Months		DTaP #4			
4–6 Years	MMR #2	DTaP #5		IPV #4	
11–18 Years		Td booster			
≥19 Years	Meningococcal[b]				

(continued)

TABLE 16–4 (Continued)

Note

- DTaP#5 is not necessary if DTaP#4 was given after the age of 4 years.

- Hep B #2 should be given 4 weeks after Hep B#1.
- Hep B #3 should be given 16 weeks after the Hep B#1 and 8 weeks after the Hep B#2.
- Hep B #3 should not be given before 6 months of age.

- Hib and PCV is not generally recommended for children aged ≥ 5 years.

- IPV is not generally for age ≥18 years.

- Td booster is given every 10 years.

[a]Varicella: Give 2 doses to all susceptible adolescent aged ≥13 years, 4 weeks apart.

[b]Meningococcal: For high risk only (asplenia, complement deficiency, college students residing in the dormitories, travelers to endemic area [Sub-Saharan Africa, Saudi Arabia])

Source with permission: CDC.gov, Department of Health and Human Services.

Combination vaccines

- Pediarix = Hep B + DTaP + IPV

- Trihibit = DTaP + Hib

- Comvax = Hep B + Hib

TABLE 16–4 (Continued)	
• ProQuad = MMR + varicella	
• Twinrix = Hep A + Hep B (approved only for age ≥ 18 years)	
• Pentavac = DTaP + IPV + Hib (note available)	
• Hexavac = DTaP + IPV + Hib + Hep B (note available)	
Immunization Injection Sites	
Intramuscular	**Subcutaneous**
• Hep B/Hep A	• MMR
• DTaP	• Varicella
• Hib	• IPV
• IPV	
• PCV	

TABLE 16–5: Well Visit Evaluation (HHIP LUV)

- Developmental milestones

- Physical examination

- Hearing

- Hb level

- Immunization status

- PPD skin testing

- Lead level

- UA → once the child is toilet trained

- Vision and hearing → after age 4 years

- After age of 10 years → ask following questions:

  1. Home environment

  2. Education

  3. Activity (extracurricular)

  4. Diet

  5. Drug use (includes tobacco, alcohol, and illicit drugs)

  6. Sexual activity (menarche in ♀)

  7. Suicidal ideation

TABLE 16–5 (Continued)

Note

- Breast milk causes seedy bowel movement.

- Infant loses weight on first 5–10 days (up to 10% of birth weight).

- Infant gains weight 1 oz/day for first 6 months.

- Baby should double weight by 6 months and triple weight by 1 year.

TABLE 16–6: Lead Management

- $<10 \rightarrow$ Only routine screening

- $10–14 \rightarrow$ Recheck every 3–4 months until two < 10 or three < 15

- $15–19 \rightarrow$ Venous confirmation within 30 days

    $\rightarrow$ Council family on abatement (must be performed by trained person)

    $\rightarrow$ Recheck every 3–4 months until two < 10 or three < 15

- $20–29 \rightarrow$ Venous confirmation within 14 days

    $\rightarrow$ If venous $> 20 \rightarrow$ refer patient to lead poisoning specialist

    $\rightarrow$ Recheck every 3–4 months until two < 10 or three < 15

- $30–39 \rightarrow$ Venous confirmation within 2 days

    $\rightarrow$ If $> 30 \rightarrow$ consider chelation Rx with BAL, succimer, or $CaNa_2$ (EDTA)

TABLE 16–7: Infections

A. Candidal oral thrush

- Nystatin susp 4–6 mL swish and swallow qid until 3 days after resolution or

- Nystatin troche 200,000–400,000 units 4–5 times per day until 3 days after resolution Or

- Mycostatin susp 100,000 units 4 drops to side of the mouth (buccal area) qid until 3 days after resolution

B. Congestion and cough

- Robitussin (see table for dosing) or

- Dimetapp or

- Triaminic or

- PediaCare

C. Diaper rash

- Mycostatin topical 100,000 units/g cream (apply topically with every change of diaper) or

- Nystatin troche 200,000–400,000 units 4–5 times per day until 3 days after resolution

TABLE 16–7 (Continued)

D. Otitis media (5 mL = 1 tsp)

- Amoxicillin 25–50 mg/kg/day PO divided tid ×
  5–10 days (suspension: 125 mg/5 mL and 250 mg/5 mL).
  High dose: 80–90 mg/kg divide bid

- If PCN allergy → azithromycin (>6 months) 10 mg/kg/
  day (max: 500 mg/day) 1 PO daily × day 1 then on
  days 2–5 give 5 mg/kg/day (max: 250 mg/day)

- If PCN allergy: consider cefuroxime 250 mg PO bid or
  suspension 30 mg/kg/day divided bid

Alternate: cefdinir, cefprozil

- If recurrent OM: give prophylaxis amoxicillin
  20 mg/kg qhs PO

- If persistent OM: augmentin, cefuroxime × 10 days or
  ceftriaxone 50 mg/kg IM single dose

(continued)

TABLE 16–7 (Continued)

E. Strep Pharyngitis (5 mL = 1 tsp)

- Penicillin V
  → If < 12 years → 250 mg PO bid–tid × 10 days 1st line

  → If ≥ 12 years → 500 mg PO bid–tid × 10 days

- Benzathine penicillin
  → If < 27 kg → 600,000 units IM × 1 dose 1st line

  → If > 27 kg → 1.2 million units IM × 1 dose

- For prevention of rheumatic fever → 1.2 million
  units IM q month, q3wk for high risk

- Amoxicillin 20–40 mg/kg PO divided tid
  (suspension: 125 mg/5 mL and 250 mg/5 mL) 1st line

- Azithromycin 12 mg/kg/day (max: 500 mg)
  PO daily × 5 days 2nd line

- Erythromycin estolate 20–40 mg/kg/day
  divided bid or tid × 10 days 2nd line

- Erythromycin ethyl succinate 40 mg/kg/day divided bid or
  qid × 10 days (max: 1 g/day) 2nd line

- Cephalexin
  → If < 1 year → 25–50 mg/kg/day PO daily 2nd line

  → If ≥ 1 year → 50–100 mg/kg/day PO daily
  (suspension: 125 mg/5 mL, 250 mg/5 mL)

TABLE 16–8: Fluid Management

Fluid Replacement

Age	Fluid Bolus (NSS/LR), 20 mL/kg	Packed Cells, 10 mL/kg
Preterm	10–20 (10 mL/kg)	10–20
Newborn	35 (10 mL/kg)	35
6 Months	140	70
1 Year	200	100
3 Years	300	140
6 Years	400	200
8 Years	500	250
10 Years	600	300

Maintenance Fluid

1st 10 kg of total body weight	100 mL/kg/day or 4 mL/kg/h
2nd 10 kg of total body weight	50 mL/kg/day or 2 mL/kg/h
>20 kg of total body weight	20 mL/kg/day or 1 mL/kg/h

Electrolyte and Caloric Requirement

- Na^+: 2–4 meq/kg/day

- K^+: 1–2 meq/kg/day

- Caloric requirement: <12 months → 100–120 kcal/kg, calorie requirement ↓ by 10 kcal/year (age 1–4)

- Adequate urinary output: 1 mL/kg/h

(continued)

TABLE 16–8 (Continued)		
Dehydration (1% = 10 mL/kg)		
Infants	**Children**	**Signs**
5% (50 mL/kg)	3% (30 mL/kg)	↑ HR (10–15% of normal)
		↓ Tear production/sweating
		Concentrated urine
		Tacky mucous membrane
10% (100 mL/kg)	6% (60 mL/kg)	As above but increase in severity
		↓ Skin turgor
		Oliguria
		Sunken fontanelle
15% (150 mL/kg)	9% (900 mL/kg)	Hypotension
		Delayed capillary refill
		Obtundation
		Kussmaul breathing

Note: If cardiovascular instability, regardless of percent of dehydration → 10–20 mL/kg isotonic fluid, follow with 10 mL/kg of blood or colloid if no response to 2 boluses.

TABLE 16–9: Gastroesophageal Reflux

Labs and Studies

• CXR PA and lateral	• Milk scan
• Salivagram	• Gastric emptying study
• pH probe study	• EGD (esophagogastroduodenoscopy)

• Upper GI series with small bowel follow through (SBFT)

Treatment

• Ranitidine (Zantac) 2–3 mg/kg bid–tid or

• Famotidine (Pepcid) 0.3–0.5 mg/kg bid or

• Cimetidine (Tagamet) 10–12.5 mg/kg qid or

• Metoclopramide (Reglan) 0.1 mg/kg qid or

• Sucralfate (Carafate)

• Surgery (Nissen fundoplication)

TABLE 16–10: Hyperkalemia Management

• Check ECG for T-wave changes

• Calcium chloride (10%) 10 mg/kg

• Insulin 0.1 mg/kg with dextrose (10–20%) 2–4 mL/kg

• Sodium bicarbonate 1–2 meq/kg

TABLE 16–11: Pertussis (Incubation Period 7–21 Days)

Signs and Symptoms

- Stage I, catarrhal (1–2 weeks): URI symptoms

- Stage II, paroxysmal (2–4 weeks): paroxysmal cough with increased severity and frequency producing characteristic whoop during the sudden forceful inspiratory phase, posttussive vomiting is also observed during this stage

- Stage III, convalescent (1–2 weeks): cough can persist for months (paroxysmal and staccato cough)

Labs and Studies

CBC with diff	CXR
Pertussis PCR and culture	Direct immunofluorescent assay of nasopharyngeal specimen

Treatment

- Erythromycin 50 mg/kg/day in 4 divided doses for 14 days can prevent progression if started in stage I

- Alternate to erythromycin: erythromycin estolate 40 mg/kg bid × 14 days

- Alternate to erythromycin: TMP–SMX but its efficacy has not been proven

- Corticosteroids and β-agonist aerosols can also be useful

TABLE 16–12: Seizure Management

- Lorazepam (Ativan) 0.05–0.1 mg /kg IV slow push or

- Diazepam (Valium) 0.1–0.3 mg/kg IV/IO, max: 1 mg/min over 5 min or 0.5 mg/kg PR initial then 0.25 mg/kg

- Phenytoin (Dilantin) 20 mg/kg IV, max dose: 1 g, max rate: 1 mg/kg/min

- Phenobarbital 20 mg/kg IV over 5 min, max dose: 1 g

Note: Benzodiazepines and phenobarbital when used concurrently can cause significant respiratory distress.

TABLE 16–13: Sepsis Workup	
Labs and Studies	
CBC with diff	CXR
Blood C&S	BMP
UA and urine C&S	PT/PTT
CSF analysis and CSF C&S	

Treatment
• Provide supplemental oxygen
• IV access
• Volume resuscitation if needed
• Patient is < 6 weeks of age: if meningitis is suspected → ampicillin or cefotaxime
• Patient is > 6 weeks of age: ceftriaxone or cefotaxime
• If penicillin-resistant meningitis is suspected → vancomycin + ceftriaxone or cefotaxime
• If *Salmonella* sepsis suspected → 3rd generation cephalosporin or TMP–SMX
• If intraabdominal focus → Unasyn or ampicillin + gentamicin + clindamycin
• If immunosuppression or central venous catheter: → nafcillin or oxacillin or dicloxacillin + vancomycin + 3rd cephalosporin

TABLE 16–14: Emergency Medications and Dosing

Name	Dose	Route	Max: Single Dose
Activated charcoal	1 g/kg	PO/NG	50 g
Adenosine	0.1 mg/kg/ 0.2 mg/kg	IV	12 mg
Albuterol	Infant: 2.5 mg Child: 5 mg	Aerosol	
Amiodarone (pulseless/VT)	5 mg/kg	IV	15 mg/kg
Atropine	0.02 mg/kg	IV/ETT	0.5 mg
Benadryl	1 mg/kg	IV/IM	50 mg
Calcium chloride (10%)	20 mg/kg	IV	500 mg
Dextrose (newborn: 10%)	5–10 mg/kg	IV	
(25%)	2–4 mg/kg	IV	
Epinephrine			
1:10,000 (0.1 mg/mL)	0.01 mg/kg	IV	
1:1000 (1 mg/kg)	0.1 mg/kg	ETT	
1:1000 (1 mg/kg)	0.01 mg/kg	Sub Q	0.35 mL

(continued)

TABLE 16–14 (Continued)			
Racemic epinephrine (Croup)	11.25 mg in 3 mL NS	Aerosol	
Nebulized epinephrine 1:1000	5 mg (5 mL)	Aerosol	
Flumazenil	0.01 mg/kg	IV	1 mg
Glucagon	<10 kg: 0.1 mg/kg	IV/IM/ Sub Q	1 mg
	>10 kg: 1 mg	IV/IM/ Sub Q	1 mg
Lasix	1 mg/kg	IV	40 mg
Lidocaine	1 mg/kg	IV/ETT	100 mg
Magnesium sulfate (500 mg/mL)	25–50 mg/kg	IV	2 g
Sodium bicarbonate (8.4%)	1 meq/kg	IV	
(Newborn: 4.2%)	2 meq/kg	IV	

17
Surgery

TABLE 17–1: Etiologies of Abdominal Pain	
RUQ	**LUQ**
Cholecystitis/cholangitis	PID in ♀
Intussusceptions	Ovarian cyst in ♀
Pancreatitis	Diverticulosis
Hepatitis/hepatomegaly	Intussusceptions
Ischemic bowel	Ischemic bowel
Bowel perforation	Bowel perforation
MI	MI
Pneumonia empyema/pleurisy	Pancreatitis
Gastritis/PUD	Pneumonia
Renal stones	Gastritis/PUD
Herpes zoster	Renal stone
Pericarditis	Herpes zoster
Retrocecal appendicitis	Splenic injury/infarct/abscess
Subdiaphragmatic abscess	Empyema
Drug screen (acetaminophen)	
Budd-Chiari syndrome	

TABLE 17–1 (Continued)	
RLQ	**LLQ**
PID in ♀	Intussusceptions
Ovarian causes ♀	Diverticulitis
Appendicitis	Ovarian causes ♀
Intussusceptions	Ischemic bowel
Ischemic colitis	Renal stone
Renal stone/nephrolithiasis	Bowel perforation
Bowel perforation	Epididymitis ♂
Epididymitis ♂	Herpes zoster
Herpes zoster	Salpingitis ♀
Salpingitis ♀	Psoas abscess
Psoas abscess	Seminal vesiculitis ♂
Seminal vesiculitis ♂	Ectopic pregnancy ♀
Ectopic pregnancy ♀	Endometriosis
Endometriosis	Inflammatory bowel disease (Crohn's or UC)
Inflammatory bowel disease (Crohn's or UC)	Irritable bowel syndrome
Irritable bowel syndrome	
Inguinal hernia	
Mesenteric adenitis	

(continued)

TABLE 17–1 (Continued)	
Epigastric	**Generalized**
Gastritis/GERD/PUD	Peritonitis
Pancreatitis	Gastroenteritis
Hernia	Bowel obstruction
MI	Fecal impaction
Pericarditis	Intestinal perforation
Ischemic bowel	Ischemic bowel Dz
Bowel perforation	Irritable bowel syndrome
Pneumonia	Porphyria
Esophageal rupture (Boerhaave's syndrome)	Metabolic/DKA/uremia
AAA rapture	Sickle cell crisis
Periumbilical	Pancreatitis
Early appendicitis	Adhesions from previous surgery
Gastroenteritis	Trauma
Bowel obstruction	Malaria
AAA rupture	Leukemia
Mesenteric adenitis	Mesenteric adenitis
Adhesions from previous surgery	Mesenteric thrombosis

TABLE 17–1 (Continued)	
Misc. Causes of Abdominal Pain	Aortic aneurysm rupture
Toxins (lead poisoning)	Sepsis
Narcotic withdrawal	Toxin
Herpes zoster	CHF
Hypersensitivity reaction	Sickle cell anemia
Acute adrenal insufficiency	Psychogenic
Henoch-Schönlein purpura	

TABLE 17–2: Initial Diagnostic Labs and Studies for Abdominal Pain

CBC with diff	BMP	Calcium and Mg level
LFT	Alk PO_4	Bilirubin
Amylase	Lipase	UA
UCG/β-HCG in ♀	Blood C&S	Urine C&S
Acute abdominal series	CT abd	US abd (mainly RUQ)
Lactic acid level (bowel infarct)	Troponin	PT/PTT/INR
Misc. Labs		
Hepatitis panel	Drug screen	Medication overdose (acetaminophen)
Clostridium difficile toxin A&B (if Abx use in past 1 month)		
Radiological Studies		

- CT (abd/pelvic): malignancy, pseudocyst, abscess, appendicitis, aortic dissection

- US: gallstones, ovarian cyst in ♀, ectopic, hydronephrosis, ascites

- CXR (pneumonia, perforation)

- Acute abdominal series/flat plate: renal stones, perforation, impaction

TABLE 17–2 (Continued)

Misc. Studies

- Colonoscopy (malignancy, inflammatory bowel disease, ischemic bowel disease)

- Upper endoscopy (gastritis, PUD)

- Upper GI series with small bowel follow through barium (malignancy, perforation)

- ERCP (stone in bile duct)

- Manual cervical examination in ♀: PID, STD (gonorrhea and chlamydia Cx, wet prep)

- Bladder scan in ♂: urinary retention (benign prostatic hypertrophy, prostate cancer)

- Laparotomy: malignancy, ovarian cyst, uterine fibroid, adhesions (Hx of previous surgery)

TABLE 17–3: Goldman Index (Risk of Major Cardiac Complication in Patient Undergoing Surgery)

Risk Factors	Points
1. Age > 70	5
2. MI in previous 6 months	10
3. S3 gallop or JVD	11
4. Important aortic stenosis	3
5. Rhythm other than sinus or premature atrial contraction on last preoperative ECG	7
6. >5 PVC/min documented in the past	7
7. PO_2 <60 or PCO_2 >50 8. K^+ < 3 or HCO_3 < 20 9. BUN > 50/Cr > 3	3
10. Abnormal AST, signs of chronic liver Dz, bedridden from noncardiac Dz	
11. Current operation → intraperitoneal, intrathoracic, or aortic operation	3
12. Emergency operation	4

Risk index: class I = 0–5 points (low), II = 6–12 (intermediate), III = 13–35 (high), IV ≥ 25 (very high)

Source with permission: Goldman L, Caldera DL, Nussbaum SR. et al. Multifactorial index of cardiac risk in noncardiac surgical procedures. *N Eng J Med* 1977;297:845–850.

TABLE 17–4: ACC/AHA Guideline: Clinical Predictor of Increased Perioperative Cardiovascular Risk

Major

- Unstable coronary syndrome
  - Acute MI (<7 days)/recent MI (7–30 days) with evidence of important ischemic risk by clinical symptoms/invasive study
  - Unstable or severe angina (Canadian class III/IV)
- Decompensated heart failure
- Significant arrhythmias
  - High-grade AV block
  - Symptomatic ventricular arrhythmias
  - Supraventricular arrhythmias with uncontrolled ventricular rate
- Severe valvular disease

Intermediate

- Mild angina (Canadian class I and II)
- Previous MI by history/pathologic Q wave
- Compensated/prior heart failure
- DM
- Renal insufficiency

TABLE 17–4 (Continued)
Minor
• Advance age
• Abnormal ECG (hypertrophy, AV blocks)
• Nonsinus rhythm
• Low functional capacity
• History of stroke
• Uncontrolled HTN

TABLE 17–5: Postoperative Fever (>100.4°F)	
Day 1–2	• Atelectasis
Day 3–5	• UTI
Day 4–7	• Infection
Day 5–7	• DVT and pulmonary embolus
Other causes	• Medications
	• Malignant hyperthermia

TABLE 17–6: Postoperative Urine Output and Ileus

- Urine output → adult → $\frac{1}{2}$ mL/kg/h

  → peds → 1 mL/kg/h

- Patient should void urine in 6–8 h, if patient does not void then consider urinary catheterization

- Postoperative Ileus → occurs 6–8 days later → check K^+ level

  → Rx → consider neostigmine

TABLE 17–7: Maintenance Fluid Requirement

First 10 kg	4 mL/kg/h	100 mL/kg/day
Second 10 kg	2 mL/kg/~~day~~ h	50 mL/kg/day
After 20 kg	1 mL/kg/~~day~~ h	20 mL/kg/day

TABLE 17–8: Yarkony–Kirk Pressure Ulcer Staging	
Stage Ia	Erythema lasting >30 min but <24 h
Stage Ib	Erythema >24 h
Stage II	Ulceration extending to dermis but not involving subcutaneous tissue
Stage III	Ulceration extending to subcutaneous tissue but not involving muscle
Stage IV	Ulceration extending to muscle but not involving bone
Stage V	Ulceration extending to bone but not involving joint space
Stage VI	Ulceration extending to joint space
Source with permission: Yarkony GM, Kirk PM, Carlson C, et al. Classification of pressure ulcers. *Arch Dermatol* 1990;126:1218.	

TABLE 17–9: Suture Classifications

Absorbable	Nonabsorbable
Catgut (plain or chromic)	Silk
Polyglycolic (Dexon)	Linen
Polyglactin (Vicryl)	Polyamide (Nylon)
Polydioxone (PDS)	Polyester (Dacron)
Polyglyconate (Maxon)	Polypropylene (Prolene)
Size	
O (largest size)	
2-O or 3-O	Skin: foot
	Deep: abdomen, back, chest
4-O	Skin: abdomen, chest, extremity, foot, scalp
	Deep: extremity, foot, scalp
5-O	Skin: abdomen, chest, eyebrow, hand, penis, scalp
	Deep: eyebrow, face, hand, lip, nose
6-O	Skin: ear, eyebrow, face, nose, penis
7-O (smallest size)	Skin: eyelid, face, lip

TABLE 17–9 (Continued)	
Suture Removal Timing	
Scalp	6–8 days
Face, eyelid, eyebrow, lip, nose	3–5 days
Ear	10–14 days
Chest	8–10 days
Abdomen	8–10 days
Extremities	12–14 days
Hand	10–14 days
Foot and sole	12–14 days
Penis	8–10 days
Note: Patients with diabetes and chronic steroid users can have delayed wound healing.	

18
ACLS

TABLE 18–1: Asystole (NR-No Response)

- Check code status
- Assess patient and check vitals
- Check the leads
- Check "ABC" (airway, breathing, circulation)
- Check pulse
- If no pulse start CPR
- Check vitals
- Consider transcutaneous pacing (TCP)
- Epinephrine 1 mg IV q3-5min
- Atropine 1 mg IV q3-5min (max: 0.04 mg/kg)
- If asystole persists: consider withholding resuscitation

Source: American Heart Association.

TABLE 18–2: A-Fib/A-Flutter (NR)

Rx for rate control

→ Diltiazem (Cardiazem) 20 mg IV over 2 min rebolus in 15 min or

→ Esmolol 500 µg/kg IV over 1 min or

→ Verapamil 2.5–5 mg IV initially then 5–10 mg IV or

→ Metoprolol (Lopressor) 50 mg PO

→ If low EF/low BP digoxin 0.5 mg IV bolus then 0.25 mg IV q2h until rate is controlled (max: 1.5 mg)

Rx for maintenance of sinus rhythm

→ Procainamide 2–6 mg/kg IV over 5 min followed by 20–80 µg/kg/min infusion (max: 2 g/day) or

→ Amiodarone (for impaired ventricular function) or

→ Ibutilide or

→ Flecainide or

→ Propafenone or

→ DC cardioversion if medical therapy fails or patient is symptomatic

Anticoagulation is recommended unless there is no contraindication

(continued)

TABLE 18–2 (Continued)

Note

- Consider anticoagulant with heparin and then coumadin.

- Urgent cardioversion: start heparin IV stat, then check transesophageal echo if no thrombosis found.

  → then cardiovert within 24 h → then anticoagulate for 4 more weeks.

- Delayed cardioversion: anticoagulate for at least 3 weeks (keep INR 2–3)

  → then cardiovert → then anticoagulate for 4 more weeks.

- Labs: BMP with Mg, TSH, CBC, troponin, cardiac echo, Holter monitoring.

TABLE 18–3: Bradycardia (NR)

- Assess patient and check vitals

- Check 12-lead ECG

- Check vitals

- If patient symptomatic → give atropine 0.5–1 mg IV push q3-5min (max: 0.04 mg/kg)

  → Then consider TCP

  → NR → dopamine 5–20 μg/kg/min

  → NR → epinephrine 2–10 μg/min

  → NR → isoproterenol 2–10 μg/min

- If ECG shows → 2nd degree type II or 3rd degree heart block → consider TCP

  → then consider placing transvenous pacemaker

- All other AV blocks → have atropine at bed site

  → When patient becomes symptomatic follow above symptomatic protocol

Note: Do not use lidocaine to treat escape slow wide complex rhythm.
Source: American Heart Association.

TABLE 18–4: Supraventricular Tachycardia (Narrow-complex Tachycardia) (NR)

- If patient is unstable → cardiovert

- Vagal maneuver/carotid massage → NR → adenosine 6 mg → NR → 12 mg → NR → 12 mg → Cardizem 15–20 mg (0.25 mg/kg) IV over 2 min → NR → after 15 min → 20–25 mg over 2 min

- Check the rhythm

- If → junctional tachycardia → can be caused by digoxin or theophylline overdose

  → If normal EF → β-blocker, Ca-blocker, amiodarone

  → If EF < 40%, CHF → amiodarone

- If → multifocal atrial tachycardia (MAT) → commonly seen in COPD patients

  → Correct hypoxemia first

  → EF → if normal → β-blocker, Ca-blocker, amiodarone

  → EF < 40%, CHF: amiodarone, diltiazem

- If → PSVT → if normal EF → β-blocker, Ca-blocker, digoxin → DC cardioversion

  → also consider procainamide, amiodarone, or sotalol

  → If EF < 40 → digoxin → NR → amiodarone → NR → diltiazem

  → If unstable → cardioversion

Source: American Heart Association.

TABLE 18–5: Ventricular Tachycardia (Wide-complex Tachycardia) Stable (NR)

- Avoid: β-blocker, Ca-blocker, digoxin

1. Monomorphic → may consider synchronized cardioversion

   A. EF < 55 → amiodarone 150 mg IV/10 min or lidocaine 0.5–0.75 mg/kg

   → then cardioversion

   B. EF > 55 → procainamide load 20 mg/min up to 17 mg/kg (1000 mg)

Then infuse 1–4 mg/min (max: 17 mg/kg)

Or

Procainamide 100 mg IV over 5 min q10min when effective, maintain IV rate at 2 mg/min

→ Also consider sotalol, amiodarone, lidocaine

2. Polymorphic → search for electrolyte abnormality (K, Mg), drug toxicity, ischemia

   A. Normal QT → if EF < 55 → amiodarone 150 mg IV/10 min or

   → Lidocaine 0.5–0.75 mg/kg

   → If EF > 55 → β-blocker, lidocaine, amiodarone, sotalol

   → NR → synchronized cardioversion

   B. Prolonged QT (suggestive of torsades) → magnesium, overdrive pacing, isoproterenol, phenytoin, lidocaine

Source: American Heart Association.

TABLE 18–6: Ventricular Fibrillation/Unstable Ventricular Tachycardia (NR)

- Start CPR (consider placing patient on ventilator)

- Precordial thump if no defibrillator immediately available

- Shock 200 J → NR → 200–300 J → 360 J

- NR → Epi 1 mg IV q3-5min or vasopressin 40 units IV × 1 dose

- NR → 360 J → NR → amiodarone 300 mg IV → then give 150 mg in 3–5 min (max: 2.2 g IV/24 h)

- NR → 360 J → lidocaine 1–1.5 mg/kg IV (may repeat in 3–5 min [max: 3 mg/kg])

- NR → 360 J → magnesium sulfate 1–2 g IV PUSH over 2 min (for hypomagnesemia/torsades de pointes)

- NR → 360 J → procainamide 30 mg/min or 100 mg IV q5min up to 17 mg/kg

- NR → 360 J → HCO_3 1 meq/kg IV

- NR → 360 J

Source: American Heart Association.

TABLE 18–7: Pulseless Electrical Activity (PEA) (NR)

- Assess patient and check vitals

- Start CPR

- Search for probable etiology; 6 Hs and 6 Ts

• Hypoxia	• Tension pneumothorax
• Hypovolemia	• Tamponade
• Hypothermia	• Thrombosis–pulmonary embolism
• Hypo or Hyperkalemia	• Thrombosis–acute coronary syndrome
• Hypo or Hyperkalemia	• Trauma
• Hydrogen ion–acidosis	• Tablets (drugs)

1. Wide QRS → possible massive myocardial injury, hyperkalemia, hypoxia, hypothermia

2. Wide QRS + slow heart → drug overdose (TCA, β-blockers, Ca-blockers, digoxin)

3. Narrow complex → consider hypovolemia, infection, PE, tamponade

- Specific causes and its treatments

1. PE → no pulse with CPR, no JVD → management: thrombolytic/surgery

2. Tension pneumothorax → no pulse with CPR, + JVD, tracheal deviation

   → Rx → needle thoracostomy

(continued)

TABLE 18–7 (Continued)

3. Cardiac tamponade → no pulse with CPR, + JVD, narrow pulse prior to arrest

> → Beck's triad (hypotension, JVD, and distant heart sounds)

> → Rx → pericardiocentesis

4. Hyperkalemia → check ECG (hyperacute T waves)

> → Rx → $CaCl$ → NR → albuterol → insulin + glucose → NR → Kayexalate

- If no etiology is found → consider the following:

> → Epinephrine 1 mg IV q3-5min → NR atropine 1 mg IV q3-5min (max: 0.04 mg/kg)

Source: American Heart Association.

TABLE 18–8: Torsades de Pointes

- Polymorphic VT plus QT prolongation (etiology of ↑ QT → see Table 2–2)

- Magnesium sulfate 1–4 g IV bolus over 5–15 min or

  Magnesium sulfate 2–20 mg/min IV infusion, max: up to 48 h until QTc interval < 440 ms

- Isoproterenol 12–20 μg/min (2 mg in 500 mL D_5W → 4 μg/mL)

- If medical treatment fails → consider ventricular pacing or cardioversion

TABLE 18–9: Wolff-Parkinson-White Syndrome (WPW)– Wide QRS Complex Tachycardia

Delta wave is negative in V_1, V_2, and aVR (+) in I, II, aVL, and aVF, and isoelectric in III

Note: Avoid → digoxin, β-blocker, Ca-blocker, and adenosine

Rx → If normal EF → DC cardioversion or

    → Amiodarone 150 mg IV over 10 min and repeat q10min or

    → Procainamide load 20 mg/min up to 17 mg/kg (1000 mg)

       then infuse 1–4 mg/min (max: 17 mg/kg) or

       Procainamide 100 mg IV over 5 min q10min

       when effective, maintain IV rate at 2 mg/min

    → Flecainide or

    → Propafenone or

    → Sotalol

Rx → If EF < 40% or CHF → DC cardioversion or

    → Amiodarone 150 mg IV over 10 min and repeat q10min

Note

- If duration of WPW > 48 h → consider anticoagulation.

- Urgent cardioversion: start heparin IV stat, then check transesophageal echo

    → then cardiovert within 24 h → then anticoagulate for 4 more weeks.

- Delayed cardioversion: anticoagulate for at least 3 weeks (keep INR 2–3)

    → then cardiovert → then anticoagulate for 4 more weeks.

Source: American Heart Association.

19
Common Calls

TABLE 19–1: Agitation/Anxiety (Behavioral Management)

- Assess patient and check vitals

- Check medication list and electrolytes

- R/O delirium (see Table 19–14)

- Haldol[a] 0.5–2 mg IV q30min or 2–5 mg IM or 0.5–2 mg PO q4-6h prn (use with caution in elderly) or

- Ativan 0.5–2 mg IV/IM/PO q6-8h prn (antidote: flumazenil 0.2 mg IV/30 s) or

- Temazepam (Restoril 7.5–30 mg PO qhs prn) (antidote: flumazenil 0.2 mg IV/30 s) or

- Hydroxyzine (Vistaril, Atarax) 50–100 mg IM/PO q6-24h prn (avoid in elderly) or

- Droperidol 0.625–2.5 mg IV or 2.5–10 mg IM (may cause Q-T prolongation) or

- Risperidone 0.5–2 mg PO and IM (prolong sedation) or

- Olanzapine (Zyprexa) 2.5–10 mg PO (prolong sedation) or

- Ziprasidone (Geodon) 10–20 mg IM (as effective as Haldol, prolong sedation) or

- Quetiapine (Seroquel) 25–100 mg PO (may cause hypotension, prolong sedation)

[a]Haldol: Start lowest dose in elderly and have Narcan 0.4–2 mg q2-3min at bedside due to respiratory depression.

TABLE 19–2: Altered Mental Status	
History	
• Check baseline mental status	• History of stroke or seizure
• Review medications	
Risk Factors of Delirium	
• Hx of cardiac, renal, hepatic disease	• Multiple medications (polypharmacy)
• Hx of psychiatric disorder	• ETOH dependence
• Hx of stroke	• Sedative dependence
• Poor nutrition	• Sleep disturbance
• Dehydration	• Recent surgery
Etiologies	
Metabolic Conditions	**Drugs**
• Hepatic encephalopathy	• Drug withdrawal
• Hypoglycemia	→ ETOH, benzodiazepines, barbiturates
• Hypoxia/hypercarbia	• Amphetamines/cocaine
• Uremia	• Antihistamines → Benadryl/Atarax
• Electrolyte disturbance	• Narcotics → Darvocet/Darvon/Demerol
→ Hyponatremia	• Benzodiazepines → Valium/Librium/Dalmane

TABLE 19–2 (Continued)	
→ Hypercalcemia/ hypocalcemia	• Steroids
→ Hypermagnesemia/ hypomagnesemia	• Anticholinergic drugs
• Acidosis	• Antiparkinsonian drugs
• Endocrinopathies	• TCA/phenothiazines/ lithium
Thyroid/parathyroid/ pituitary	• Anticonvulsants
• Vitamin deficiencies	→ Phenytoin/ Phenobarbital/ Valproic acid
B_{12}/folate/thiamine	• Antimicrobials
• Toxins → CO/lead/ mercury/manganese	→ 3rd and 4th generation cephalosporins
• Porphyria	→ Acyclovir, amphotericin B, quinines, INH
Infectious	→ Rifampin
• Meningitis	• CV drugs
• Encephalitis	→ β-Blocker/digoxin/ clonidine
• Abscess	• Antineoplastic drugs
• Neurosyphilis	• Immunosuppressive agents
• Systemic infection	
• Bacteremia/Sepsis	

(continued)

TABLE 19–2 (Continued)	
Neurologic	**Miscellaneous**
• Stroke/TIA	• CHF and other cardiovascular causes
• Seizure	• Perioperative
• Head trauma	Anesthesia/drug
• Hypertensive encephalopathy	Anemia
• Malignancy	Embolism
• Migraine	Hypotension
• Vasculitis	Fluid shift/electrolyte disturbance
• Limbic encephalitis	• Dehydration
	• Sleep deprivation
	• Depression
Complete Physical Examination	
• Monitor BP, pulse, RR, temp	• O$_2$ saturation
• Observe general appearance	• Look for signs of local and systemic infection
• Mini-mental status examination	• Look for signs of meningitis
• Detail neurological examination	• Look for signs of liver disease

TABLE 19–2 (Continued)	
Activity	Quiet room, daily orientation, fall precaution
Dx studies	Labs: CBC with diff, CMP, Mg, Ca, B_{12}, folate, thiamine, TSH, VDRL/RPR, UA, troponin
	Radiological studies: CXR, CT with and without contrast, abdominal flat plate, MRI
	Special tests: ECG, ammonia, ABG, drug screen, UA C&S, blood C&S, LP, EEG, PTH

Management

- Perform mini-mental status examination

• Sitter	• Control noise stimulation
• Geri-chair	• Sleep management
• Low bed	• Reorientation

Modalities for Safety and Controlling Agitation

- Restraint
  (Posey west, 4-point restraint only in severe cases) or

- Haldol 0.5–2 mg IV or 2–5 mg IM or 0.5–2 mg PO q30min (see max dose) or

- Ativan 0.5–2 mg IV q6h 0.5–2 mg sublingual q30min (see max dose) or

- Risperdal 0.5–1 mg PO bid or

- Olanzapine 2.5–5 mg

TABLE 19–3: High Blood Pressure

- Assess patient and check vitals

- Review H&P

- Review medications

Life-threatening Conditions	Signs and Symptoms
• Hypertensive encephalopathy	• HA, blurry vision
• MI	• Chest pain (may not have chest pain in elderly/DM)
• Aortic dissection	• Back pain, chest pain
• Neuro	• Sensory or motor loss, altered mental status
• Arterial thrombus	• Peripheral pulses
• Renal	• Decrease urine output
• Eclampsia in pregnancy	• Seizure, convulsions

TABLE 19–4: Blood Pressure Classification				
	High BP	**Urgency**	**Emergency**	
BP	>180/110	>180/110	>220/140	
Si/Sx	Headache	Severe headache	Chest pain, SOB (shortness of breath)	
	Anxiety	SOB	Dysarthria	
	Asymptomatic	Edema	Altered consciousness	
			Encephalopathy	
			Pulmonary edema	
			CVA	
			Cardiac ischemia	

TABLE 19–5: BP Management (IV Management)

IV Agents	Dosage	Onset	Duration
Nitroprusside	Drip 50 mg in 250 mL D_5W start at 3 µg/kg/min; max: 10 µg/kg/min (check thiocyanate level) Caution: If used > 24 h especially in renal failure	Seconds	3–5 min
Esmolol	5 g in 500 mL D_5W, loading dose of 500 µg/kg over 1 min then 50–200 µg/kg/min	1–2 min	10–30 min
Trimethaphan	0.5–5 mg/min (useful in aortic dissection)	1–3 min	10 min
Nicardipine	5 mg/h, increase by 1–2.5 mg/h q15min, max: 15 mg/h	1–5 min	3–6 h
Nitroglycerin	0.25–5 µg/kg/min, may develop tolerance	2–5 min	3–5 min
Fenoldopam	0.1–1.6 µg/mg/min, may protect renal fx.	4–5 min	<10 min

TABLE 19–5 (Continued)			
Hydralazine	5–20 mg q20min IV (SE: headache)	10–30 min	2–6 h
Labetalol	Start at 20 mg IV → 40 mg → 60 mg → 80 mg; repeat every 10–15 min, max: 300 mg	5–10 min	3–6 h
Furosemide	10–80 mg IV (use in conjunction with vasodilator)	15 min	4 h
Enalapril (Vasotec)	1.25 mg q6h IV (max: 5 mg/24 h), may continue as PO contra-indications: Cr > 3 or renal stenosis	15 min	>6 h

TABLE 19–6: BP Management (Oral Agents)			
PO Agents	**Dosage**	**Onset**	**Duration**
Clonidine	0.1–0.2 mg PO initially then 0.1 mg q1h up to 0.8	30–60 min	6–8 h
Captopril	12.5—25 mg PO tid (may cause hypotension)	15–30 min	4–6 h
Nifedipine	10 mg PO, may repeat after 30 min (tid)	15 min	2–6 h
Labetalol	200–400 mg PO q2-3h	30 min–2h	2–12 h
Prazosin	1–2 mg PO q1h	1–2h	8–12 h

TABLE 19–7: Low Blood Pressure

- Assess patient and check vitals

- Review H&P

- Place patient in Trendelenburg position

- Check current medications
  (antihypertensive medication, Reglan, SSRI, TCA)

- Check pulse → if bradycardia < 60 → check 12-lead ECG

- Check oxygen saturation

- Check stool guaiac for any blood loss

- If blood loss suspected → type and screen at least
  2 units PRBC

- Check CBC, BMP, Mg level, PT/PTT
  (low K^+ can impair pressor response)

- Consider transfer to unit

- Rx: → NS or LR → keep wide open

  → If still hypotensive consider transferring to the unit

  → Consider starting patient on norepinephrine and
    dopamine drip (see below)

- Epinephrine (Levophed): ACLS dosing range:
  0.5–30 µg/min or

  - Mix 4 mg in 500 mL D_5W

  - Initially → 4 µg/min = 30 mL/h; usual range →
    8–12 µg/min

(continued)

TABLE 19-7 (Continued)

- Microgram to mL comparison according to mixture of 4 mg in 500 mL

  1. 4 μg/min = 30 mL/h

  2. 6 μg/min = 45 mL/h

  3. 8 μg/min = 60 mL/h

  4. 10 μg/min = 75 mL/h

- Dopamine dosing:
  (max: 50 μg/kg/min); starts at >15 μg/kg/min

  - Premixed in D_5W → 0.8 mg/mL in 250 mL or 500 mL

    → 1.6 mg/mL in 250 mL or 500 mL

    → 3.2 mg/mL in 250 mL

- Transfer patient to the unit

Work-up for Low Blood Pressure		
• CBC with diff	• Amylase	• Troponin
• BMP	• Lipase	• ABG
• ECG	• LFT	• Tox. screen
• Fibrinogen	• Lactate level	• CXR
• Fibrin split products	• UA	• Abdominal x-ray (R/O obstruction)

TABLE 19–8: Bradycardia (<60), NR-No Response

- Generally, there is no need to treat unless the patient is symptomatic

- Assess patient and check vitals

- Ask for any symptoms: lightheadedness/dizziness/syncope/palpitation/SOB/CP

- Meds (especially β-blocker, Ca^+ channel blocker—hold meds)

- Check ECG → check for any pause, blocks

- See Table 18-3

- If sinus pause → if < 2.5 s and asymptomatic → no Rx needed

  → If 2.5–3 s and asymptomatic → atropine/Epi/dopamine

  → If NR → external pacer (TCP) (see below for dosing)

  → If > 3 s and asymptomatic → requires external pacer

- Atropine 0.5–1 mg IV q3-5min (max: 0.04 mg/kg) or

- Dopamine 5–20 µg/kg/min or

- Epinephrine 2–10 µg/min

TABLE 19–9: Chest Congestion

- Humibid LA 1–2 tab q12h, 600–1200 mg q12h or

- Guaifenesin 100–400 mg PO q4h or 600–1200 mg PO q12h or

- Pseudoephedrine 60 mg PO q4h

- Chest PT (flutter)

TABLE 19–10: Chest Pain

- Assess patient and check vitals

- Define pain: site/description/intensity (1–10)/radiation/associated symptoms (N/V)

- Quick med Hx (recent surgery, cardiac risks[a])

- Life-threatening conditions → MI/PE/aortic dissection/tension pneumo/tachyarrhythmia

- Other conditions → GERD/esophageal spasm/zoster/costochondritis/anxiety

- Physical examination: cardiovascular and pulmonary

- If MI suspected → consider transferring patient to unit

- Labs: CBC with diff, BMP, Mg, troponin level, CXR, spiral CT, abdominal CT, tox. screen

- Management: → 2 L O_2 via nasal cannula (R/O tension pneumothorax by auscultation)

- If MI is suspected

  → 12-lead ECG (compare with previous ECG)

  → 0.4 mg sublingual nitroglycerin × 3 q5min → if chest pain continues → morphine 2–4 mg IV
  Note: Hold nitro if SBP < 90 or pulse < 50.

TABLE 19–10 (Continued)

→ ASA 325 mg crushed
→ Troponin × 3 (1st now and every 8 h), CPK MB q8h × 24 h
→ If pain is not relieved by nitro or morphine, consider Maalox 30 mL or GI cocktail
→ If documented MI (see Table 2–12)
• If GERD is suspected → consider Maalox 30 mL or Pepto-Bismol 30 mL
• Suspect PE in recent Hx. of major surgery → venous Doppler of LE, spiral CT or V-Q scan
• If pneumothorax is suspected: check CXR
• Suspect aortic dissection → if back pain and ↑ BP → check abdominal CT
[a]Cardiac risks: (+) FH, age, gender, DM, HTN, obesity, dyslipidemia, smoker.

TABLE 19–11: Constipation Management

Bulk laxative

- Psyllium (Metamucil, Perdiem, Fiberall)

- Methylcellulose (Citrucel)

- Polycarbophil (FiberCon, Equalactin, Konsyl Fiber)

Examples

  - Bran powder 1–4 tbs bid; onset >24 h

  - Psyllium 1 tsp daily-bid; onset >24 h

  - Methylcellulose 1 tsp daily–bid; onset >24 h

Osmotic laxative

- Magnesium hydroxide (Milk of Magnesia)

- Magnesium citrate (Evac–Q–Mag)

- Sodium phosphate
  (Fleet Enema, Fleet Phospho-Soda, Visicol)

Example

  - Mg hydroxide/Mg sulfate 20–30 mL daily–bid; onset 3–12 h

  - Sodium phosphate 45 mL in 12 oz H_2O, may repeat in 10 h, prior to colonoscopy; onset 1–6 h

Poorly absorbed sugar

- Lactulose (Cephulac, Chronulac, Duphalac)

- Sorbitol (Cytosol)

- Mannitol

TABLE 19–11 (Continued)

- Polyethylene glycol and electrolytes (Colyte, GoLYTELY, NuLYTELY)

- Polyethylene glycol (Miralax)

Example

- Sorbitol 70% 30–60 mL daily–tid; onset 24–48 h

- Lactulose 30–60 mL daily–tid; onset 24–48 h

- Polyethylene glycol (PEG) 4 L PO administer over 2–4 h, useful prior to colonoscopy; onset <4 h

Stimulant laxative

- Cascara sagrada (Colamin, Sagrada-lax)

- Castor oil (Purge, Neoloid, Emulsoil)

- Bisacodyl (Dulcolax, Correctol)

- Sodium picosulfate (Lubrilax, Sur-lax)

- Docusate sodium (Colace, Regulax, SS, Surfax)

- Mineral oil (Fleet Mineral Oil)

Example

- Bisacodyl 5–15 mg PO; onset 6–8 h

- Bisacodyl 10 mg PR; onset 1 h

- Cascara 4–8 mL/2 tab; onset 8–12 h

- Senna 5–15 mg (max: 3 × daily) (useful in constipation due to narcotic use; onset 8–12 h)

(continued)

TABLE 19–11 (Continued)

Rectal enema/suppository

- Phosphate enema (Fleet Enema)

- Mineral oil retention enema (Fleet Mineral Oil Enema)

- Tap water enema

- Soapsuds Enema

- Glycerin bisacodyl suppository

Example

- Tap water enema 500 mL PR till clear; onset 5–15 min

- Phosphate enema 120 mL PR; onset 5–15 min
  (useful for acute constipation)

- Soapsuds enema up to 1500 mL PR; onset 5–15 min
  (can cause mucosal damage)

Cholinergic agent

- Bethanechol (Ure cholic)

- Colchicine (Colsalide)

- Misoprostol (Cytotec)

Prokinetic agent

- Cisapride[a] (Propulsid)

- Tegaserod (Zelnorm)

[a]This drug is only available through limited-access program
(by Janssen Pharmaceutical and FDA).

TABLE 19–12: Cough/Throat Irritation

- Robitussin/Dimetapp 10 mL q4h prn, if congestion → Robitussin DM 10 mL q4hprn or

- Tessalon Perles 100–200 mg PO tid or

- Cepacol lozenges/spray prn (also comes in sugar free, good for diabetics) or

- Chloraseptic lozenges prn

Note: Avoid Robitussin/Dimetapp in patient with HTN.

TABLE 19–13: Death (Pronouncing Death)

- When called to pronounce death, check the following:

  1. Respiration (should be absent)

  2. Pulse (should be absent)

  3. Pupillary reaction (should be fixed and dilated)

  4. Reaction to pain stimuli → sternal rub (should be absent)

- Document above being absent/present as well as date and time of examination

- Inform family member and primary care physician about the death

- Notify family member and ask family about having an autopsy performed

- Document probable cause of death

- Inform coroner if necessary

- Sign a death certificate

- See Table 20–11 for how to write a death note

TABLE 19–14: Delirium

- Assess patient

- Check vitals (BP, pulse, respiration, temp), O_2 saturation, and I/O

Check Current Medications
(examples of medication that can cause delirium)

• Atarax	• Darvocet	• Librium
• Benadryl	• Darvon	• Valium
• Dalmane	• Demerol	• Vistaril

Labs to Order

• CBC	• Troponin I	• ECG
• CMP	• UA	• CXR
• BGM	• Tox. screen	• Urine C&S

Management

1. Sitter

2. Geri-chair

3. Low bed, bed alarm

4. Environmental changes

   - Keep windows open at daytime; have sun light exposure

   - Keep a clock and a calendar in the room for orientation

   - Make sure patient wears glasses and hearing aids while awake

TABLE 19–14 (Continued)

5. Make sure patient is well hydrated
   (be cautious in heart failure patients)

6. Restraint (Posey west, 4-point in extreme cases)

7. Haldol 0.5–2 mg IV q30 min or 2–5 mg IM or
   0.5–2 mg PO or

8. Ativan 0.5–2 mg PO sublingual q30 min or

9. Olanzapine 2.5–5 (max: 15 mg/day) PO daily or

10. Risperidone 0.5 mg PO bid (max: 6 mg/day in elderly),
    may cause hypotension or

11. Quetiapine 25 mg PO bid (max: 800 mg/day) or

12. Clozapine 12.5 mg PO bid (max: 450 mg/day), may cause
    agranulocytosis or

13. Ziprasidone 20 mg PO bid (max: 80 mg/day) or
    10–20 mg IM bid (max: 40 mg/day)

TABLE 19–15: Diarrhea

If etiology is infectious: check stool leukocytes, ova, parasite, and culture, Hep A IgM and IgG

If etiology is antibiotic induced: check stool for *Clostridium difficile* toxin A and B

- Fluid replacement

- Kaopectate 1200–1500 mg PO after loose bowel movement (BM) or

- Imodium 2 caps PO initially or

- Lomotil 2 tab or 10 mL PO qid or

- Metamucil 1–2 tab with juice or

- Carafate 1 g PO 1 h prior to meal and qhs

TABLE 19–16: Dizziness

- Assess patient and check vitals

- BGM → low (50–60) → give orange juice → if < 50 → 1 amp of glucose $D_{50}W$ (1 amp of $D_{50}W$ can ↑ glucose by 100)

- Check meds

- BP and pulse (check orthostasis)

  - (Orthostasis: ↑ in pulse of >10 bpm or ↓ 20 mmHg SBP when patient changes from recumbent to an erect position (usually occurs when 15–20% of fluid has been lost)

- Perform fecal occult blood test to R/O GI bleed

- Check 12-lead ECG to R/O arrhythmia

- Check electrolytes

- Studies to consider: echo, Holter monitor, tilt table, CT/MRI, carotid Doppler tilt table

TABLE 19–17: Dry Nose

- Ocean spray nasal spray or

- Saline nasal spray

TABLE 19–18: Dyspepsia/Heartburn

- Maalox 30 mL PO or Pepto-Bismol 30 mL or Mylanta 30 mL PO or Amphojel 30 mL PO

- Prilosec 20 mg PO daily (PPI) or Protonix 40 mg PO daily (PPI) or H_2 blocker or

- Reglan 10 mg 30 min prior to meal or

- GI cocktail → Maalox or Mylanta 30 mL + viscous lidocaine (2%) 10 mL + Donnatal 10 mL

TABLE 19–19: End of Life (Management of Patient with Dyspnea)

Mild	Severe	Critically Ill
• Hydrocodone 5 mg q4h or	• Morphine 5–15 mg q4h or	Morphine or fentanyl infusion
• Codeine 30 mg q4h; patient can be given q2h for breakthrough doses	• Oxycodone 5–10 mg q4h	

Source with permission: Mosenthal AC. *J Am Coll Surg* 2002; V194:381. American College of Surgeons.

TABLE 19–20: Epistaxis

- Assess patient and check vitals

- Have patient lean forward to avoid swallowing blood

- Apply pressure distal part of nose

- Next step → chemical cautery: silver nitrate, trichloroacetic acid

- Next step → nasal packing

- Next step → Epistat catheter

- Next step → Epistat II™ catheter

- Next step → Merocel nasal tampon

- Check CBC with diff and PT/PTT

TABLE 19–21: Fall

- Assess patient and check vitals

- Stabilize patient (ABCs) and assess patient for injury

- Check medication list
  (also check medication list that causes delirium)

- Ask current symptoms
  (dizziness, lightheadedness, headache, weakness)

- Search for etiology and treat appropriately

- Consider restraint chemical or physical restraint
  (Haldol, Posey) (also see Tables 19–1 and 19–14)

TABLE 19–22: Fever (Temp > 100.4°F)

- If first episode → investigate etiology

- Consider acetaminophen (Tylenol) 650 mg PO 1 tab × 1 now

- Consider cooling blanket: D/C when temp ≤ 102.5°F

- Assess for phlebitis, Foley, IV and art lines, decubitus ulcer, skin breakdown, rash

- Check previous CBC, CXR, cultures

- Suspicion of sepsis → order CBC with diff, UA, urine R&M, urine C&S, stool C&S, blood C&S × 2 15 min apart from 2 different sites, stool *C. difficele* toxin A&B

Also consider CXR (AP and lateral), sputum C&S and acid-fast stain

TABLE 19–23: GI Bleed

- Assess patient

- Check vitals:
  BP (orthostasis if patient is dizzy or lightheaded), pulse

- Symptoms:
  lightheadedness/dizziness/syncope/ palpitation/SOB

- Medical Hx of → PUD, hemorrhoids, diverticulosis

- Check meds (heparin, warfarin, ASA, Plavix, NSAID)

- To determine upper or lower GI bleed → place NG tube

- Hb/Hct q2-6h

- PT/PTT/INR/platelets

TABLE 19–24: Glucose (High)

- Assess patient and check vitals

- Check med list

- Give insulin[a] according to sliding scale

- Check patient's last insulin/antihyperglycemic med/other meds

- Check for patient's diet status

- Search for etiology: medications (e.g., steroids)

Blood Sugar[a]	Sub Q Regular Insulin(Units)
150–200	2
201–250	4
251–300	6
301–350	8
351–400	10
401–450	12

- If >400 → check urine ketones, serum ketone, and BMP (serum ketone measures only acetoacetate)

    → Check for serum β-hydroxybutyrate

- Recheck blood sugar in 45 min–1 h after giving insulin (see Table 4–3)

[a]Insulin sliding scale may vary from institution to institution.

TABLE 19–25: Glucose (Low)

- Assess patient and check vitals

- Check for symptoms
  (sweating, tachycardia, dizziness, weakness)

- If between 50 and 60 → give orange juice with crackers

- If symptomatic or <50 → 1 amp of glucose $D_{50}W$
  (1 amp can ↑ glucose by 100)

- If no IV access → glucagon 1 mg IM
  (SE: nausea/vomiting)

- Check blood sugar every 30 min to every hour until stable

TABLE 19–26: Headache

- Assess patient and check vitals

- Check meds (nitro)

- Recent procedure (spinal tap, epidural)

- Check for focal neurological deficits

- Consider CT or MRI of head if intracerebral pathology suspected

- Rx: low flow O_2

1. Tylenol 650 mg PO × 1 now
   (check LFT; if high, consider alternative) or

2. NSAIDS: ibuprofen 600 mg PO
   (check LFT; if high, consider alternative)

3. Antiemetics

4. Narcotics (if no response to above modalities)

5. Triptans or ergots for migraine headache
   (be cautious in HTN)

TABLE 19–27: Hiccups

- Assess patient and check vitals
- Baclofen: 10–20 mg IV q8h (1st line)
- Chlorpromazine (Thorazine) 25–50 mg PO/IM q6h 2nd line
- Metoclopramide 5–10 mg q6-8h 2nd line
- Phenergan 10 mg PO q6h 2nd line
- Nifedipine 10–20 mg daily–tid 2nd line
- Amitriptyline 10 mg PO tid 2nd line
- Haloperidol 2–10 mg IM 2nd line

TABLE 19–28: Laceration

- Assess patient and check vitals

Immunization Status	Clean, Minor Wound		All Other Wound	
	Td	TIG	Td	TIG
≥3 Doses received in immunization series	Give only if last booster >10 years	No	If last booster >5 years	No[a]
<3 Doses received or uncertain of immunization	Yes	No	Yes	Yes

- Tetanus toxoid dosage 0.5 mg IM × 1 dose
- Td and TIG should be given on two separate sites

Abbreviations: TIG, tetanus immunoglobulin; Td, tetanus toxoid.
[a]TIG is not given unless patient has humoral immune deficiency (e.g., HIV and agammaglobulinemia).
Source with permission: MMWR Morb Mortal wkly Rep 40(RR-10):1, 1991.

TABLE 19–29: Nausea

- Phenergan 12.5–25 mg IV/PO/IM/PR q4-6h or

- Compazine 5–10 mg IV over 2 min, 5–10 mg PO/IM tid–qid, 25 mg supp PR bid or

- Zofran 8 mg PO bid (if >12 years), 4 mg PO tid (if <12 years) or

- Tigan 250 mg PO q6-8h, 200 mg IM/PR q6-8h or

- Reglan 10 mg IV/IM q2-3h, 10–15 mg PO qid 30 min before meal (recommended for patient with GI dysmotility)

TABLE 19–30: Pain Management

Note: Patient with DNR status → be liberal with pain medication when managing pain

Do not give meperidine (Demerol) with MAOI → it can kill a patient

- Assess pain and document
  (location, intensity, quality, severity)

- Consider increasing pain med dose if the patient is already on pain med

- Search for etiology of pain → consider treating the cause of pain

- Be cautious of using opiates in patient with hypotension

Mild–moderate pain

- Tylenol 325–650 mg PO/PR q4-6 h (max: 4 g/24 h) or

- Tylenol # 3 (codeine + acetaminophen [30/300]) 1–2 tab PO q4-6h or

- Tylenol with codeine elixir 15 mL q4-6h or

- Salicylate → aspirin 325–650 mg PO/PR q4-6h or

  → salsalate 500–750 mg PO q8-12h or

- Propionic acids → ibuprofen 200–600 mg PO q4-6 or

  → naproxen 250–500 mg PO bid or

- Acetic acids → sulindac 150–200 mg PO bid or

  → diclofenac 50 mg PO bid–tid, 75 mg PO bid

(continued)

TABLE 19–30 (Continued)

Moderate pain

- Acetic acids → ketorolac (Toradol) 10 mg PO q4-6h, 15–30 mg IM/IV q6h (max: 5 days) or

- Opioid agonist → codeine 0.5–1 mg/kg (15–60 mg PO/IM/IV/Sub Q q4-6h prn, oral solution 15 mg/5 mL

  → Propoxyphene 65–100 mg PO q4h prn or

  → Meperidine (Demerol) 1–1.8 mg/kg IM/Sub Q or slow IV q3-4h (max: 150 mg)

  → 50–150 mg PO q3-4h prn

  → 75 mg IV/IM/Sub Q = 300 mg, tab = 50,100 mg; syrup = 50 mg/5 mL

- Opioid combo → Darvocet (propoxyphene + acetaminophen [50/325]) 2 tab PO q4h prn or

  → Lortab (hydrocodone + acetaminophen [2.5/500]) 1–2 tab PO q4-6h prn or

  → Percocet (oxycodone + acetaminophen [2.5/325]) 1–2 tab PO q6h prn or

  → Percodan (oxycodone + ASA [5/325]) 1 tab PO q6h prn or

  → Vicodin (hydrocodone + acetaminophen [5/500]) 1–2 tab PO q4-6h prn

- Opioid agonist–antagonist → pentazocine (Talwin) 30 mg IV/IM q3-4h prn or

  → Talwin NX (pentazocine + naloxone [50/0.5]) 1 tab PO q3-4h prn or

TABLE 19–30 (Continued)

→ Butorphanol (Stadol) 0.5–2 mg IV or 1–4 mg IM q3-4h prn or
→ Butorphanol (Stadol) 1 spray (1 mg) in 1 nostril q3-4h prn
• Other → tramadol (Ultram) 50–100 mg PO q4-6h prn
(Seizure can occur with concurrent use of antidepressants and patient with Hx. of seizure disorder)

Moderate–severe pain

• Morphine 1–2 mg (max: 15 mg) IM/Sub Q or slow IV q4h prn or
• MS Contin 30 mg PO q8-12h or
• Opioid agonist
→ Meperidine (Demerol) 1–1.8 mg/kg IM/Sub Q or slow IV q3-4h (max: 150 mg) or
→ 50–150 mg PO q3-4h prn
→ Tab = 50,100 mg; syrup = 50 mg/5 mL
• Hydromorphone (Dilaudid) 2–4 mg PO q4-6h prn or
→ 0.5–2 mg IM/Sub Q or slow IV q4-6h prn
• Fentanyl (transdermal patch [Duragesic, Actiq]) 25–100 μg/h (see Table 19–32)

Note

• 1 mg Dilaudid = 7 mg morphine, 1 mg morphine = 7 mg Demerol
• Allergy to codeine → give Darvocet
• Darvocet is known to cause delirium in elderly.

TABLE 19–31: Pain Meds, Onset of Action and Dosing Equivalents Between PO and IV				
Medication	**Onset (Min)**	**Dosing (H)**	**Oral (mg)**	**IV (mg)**
			Equivalents	
Codeine	10–30	4	200	120
Hydromorphone (Dilaudid)	15–30	4	7.5	1.5
Levorphanol (Levo-dromoran)	30–90	4	4	2
Meperidine (Demerol)	10–45	4	300	75
Methadone	15–60	4	30	10
Morphine (Roxanol)	15–60	4	30	10
Morphine CR (MS Contin)	15–60	12	90	
Oxycodone CR (Oxycontin)	15–30	12	30	
Propoxyphene	30–60	4	200	

TABLE 19-32: Fentanyl Patch Dosing Compared to Other Narcotics (1 mg = 1000 µg)[a]

Fentanyl 25µg/h

	PO/day	IM/day	50 µg/h		75 µg/h	
			PO/day	IM/day	PO/day	IV/day
Codeine (Tylenol + codeine)	150–447	104–286	448–747	287–481	748–1047	482–676
Oxycodone (Percocet)	22.5–67	12–33	67.5–112	33.1-56	112.5–157	56.1-78
Morphine	45–134	8–22	135–224	23–37	225–314	38–52
Hydromorphone (Dilaudid)	5.6–17	1.2–3.4	17.1–28	3.5–5.6	28.1–39	5.7–7.9

Fentanyl 100 µg/h

	PO/day	IV/day	125 µg/h		150 µg/h	
			PO/day	IV/day	PO/day	IM/day
Codeine (Tylenol + codeine)	1048–1347	677–871	1348–1647	872–1066	1648–1947	1067–1261
Oxycodone (Percocet)	157–202	78.1–101	202.5–247	101.1–123	247.5–292	123.1–147
Morphine	315–404	53–67	405–494	68–82	495–548	83–97
Hydromorphone (Dilaudid)	39.1–51	8–10	51.1–62	10.1–12	62.1–73	12.1–15

[a]The patch takes 16 h to take effect.

TABLE 19–33: Sinus Pause

- Assess patient and check vitals

  → If <2.5 seconds and asymptomatic → no Rx needed

  → If 2.5–3 seconds and asymptomatic → atropine then Epi/dopamine

  → External pacer at bed site

  → If >3 seconds and asymptomatic → requires pacer placement

  → If symptomatic → requires pacer placement

- Atropine 0.5–1 mg IV q3-5min (max: 0.04 mg/kg)

- Epinephrine 2–10 µg/min

- Dopamine 5–20 µg/kg/min

TABLE 19–34: Sleep Disturbance/Insomnia

- Temazepam (Restoril) 7.5 mg PO qhs or

- Zolpidem (Ambien) 5 mg PO qhs
  (good for patient requiring less sedation) or

- Trazodone (Desyrel) 50–100 mg PO qhs
  (use 25 mg in elderly) or

- Alprazolam (Xanax) 0.25 mg PO qhs
  (avoid in elderly or patient with delirium) or

- Benadryl 25–50 mg PO qhs
  (avoid in elderly or patient with delirium) or

- Sonata 10–20 mg PO qhs
  (half the dose in elderly and liver disease)

Some medications may cause confusion or dizziness.

TABLE 19–35: Shortness of Breath[a]

- Assess patient

- Check vitals

- Ask for associated symptoms
  (think of the following—MI, PE, Pneumo)

- Medical Hx. (e.g., COPD) → do not give high flow
  O_2 (<2 L O_2)

- Order: troponin, ABG, O_2 sat, spiral CT

- Stat ECG, CXR, CBC with diff, CMP

- Physical examination: lungs → crackles/rhonchi

- Suspicion of possible CHF → give Lasix 40 mg IV
  (can be repeated)

- Suspicion of COPD → low flow O_2 (max: 2 L O_2)

  → Solu-medrol 40–80 mg IV q6-8h

- Wheezing/rhonchi → breathing Tx (DuoNeb/albuterol)

- Suspect PE → if recent Hx. of surgery, oral contraceptive
  use, hypercoagulable state, immobilized

- Give 2 L O_2 → 4 L → 6 L and check sat

- If patient doesn't respond to 6 L of oxygen → call
  respiratory therapist

  → give 40% Venti mask → check ABG in 1/2 h

  → 100% nonrebreather mask → check ABG in 1/2 h

  → BIPAP–Settings → I/E (14/6) → check ABG in 1/2 h

Note: I = ventilation, E = oxygenation.

(continued)

TABLE 19–35 (Continued)
→ Do not leave patient with COPD on high conc. O_2 for long time, it can cause respiratory depression
→ Intubate: TV: 7–10 mL/kg → check ABG in $1/2$ h, RR: 12–18, FiO_2: 100% → 80% → 60%
→ See Table 3–13 for ventilator setting
• Sometimes albuterol breathing Rx can cause tachycardia → use Xopenex 0.6–1.25 mg q6-8h
[a]1 L of NC can ↑ O_2 sat by 3%, room air has 21% O_2.

TABLE 19–36: Syncope
(Loss of Consciousness for Brief Period)

Etiology	
Neurally Mediated	**Orthostatic**
Vasovagal	Drug induced (see list below)
Carotid sinus syndrome	Autonomic nervous system failure
Situational (cough/postmicturition)	→ DM, ETOH, amyloid, parkinsonism
Cardiopulmonary Conditions	**Cardiac Arrhythmia**
MI	Sick sinus
Aortic dissection	AV block
Pericardial tamponade/dz.	SVT/VT
Pulmonary emboli	WPW/torsades de pointes
Aortic stenosis	**Neurologic**
HOCM	TIA
Pulmonary HTN	Seizure
Medication Induced	Migraine
• Diuretics/Vasodilators	**Psychogenic**
• Q-T elongating drugs	Anxiety
Quinidine, procainamide, disopyramide	Hyperventilation

(continued)

TABLE 19–36 (Continued)	
Sotalol, ibutilide, dofetilide, amiodarone	**Other**
Phenothiazines	Metabolic (glucose)
Amitriptyline, imipramine, Geodon	Anemia (bleed)
Erythromycin, pentamidine, fluconazole	ETOH use
Astemizole	Cataplexy
Droperidol	Acute hypoxemia

Syncope management

- Assess patient and check vitals

- BGM → low (<60) → see Table 19–25

- Check meds

- BP and pulse (orthostasis)

  → Orthostasis: ↑ in pulse of >10 bpm or ↓ 20 mmHg systolic BP when patient changes from recumbent to an erect position (usually occurs 15–20% of fluid has been lost)

- If bleeding is suspected → perform fecal occult blood test

- If arrhythmia is suspected → check 12-lead ECG

- Order BMP

- Possible positional/vasovagal

Diagnostic studies

Labs/studies: CBC with diff, CMP, Ca, Mg, TSH, troponin, CXR, CT/MRI
Special tests: ECG, Holter, echo, carotid Doppler, EEG, head-up tilt, drug screen, ABG

TABLE 19–37: Tachycardia (>100)[a]

- Assess patient and check vitals

- Check temp (a high temp can cause tachycardia)

- Ask for any symptoms:
  lightheadedness/dizziness/syncope/palpitation/SOB/CP

- Check ECG → check for arrhythmia
  (see Chapter 2 for management)

- Review medications and search for etiology

- Manage appropriately

[a]Also see Chapter 2 for arrhythmia.

TABLE 19–38: Unresponsive Patient[a]

- Check code status

- ABCs

- Assess patient, check vitals, and O_2 sat

- BGM → low (<55) → thiamine 10 mg IV + 1 amp of glucose $D_{50}W$ (1 amp → ↑ glucose by 100)

- Cardiac rhythm (12-lead ECG) → look for arrhythmia, blocks, and MI

- CMP (Chem 12) plus Mg

- Urine tox or serum tox

- If morphine/other narcotic induced

  → Give Narcan 0.2–2 mg IV/IM/Sub Q q5min

- If benzodiazepine induced → flumazenil 0.2 mg IV over 30 s

  → Follow by → 0.3 mg IV at 1 min → 0.5 mg IV at 2 min

Note

- Flumazenil can cause seizure in patient who is on benzodiazepines chronically.

- Flumazenil is contraindicated in hepatic encephalopathy.

- Flumazenil may not be effective in chronic benzodiazepine users.

[a]Also see Tables 19–2 and 19–14.

20
Writing Notes

TABLE 20–1: Admission Orders: Time and Date

- Admit to: team, unit, attending

- Diagnosis: working diagnosis

- Condition: stable/critical/guarded

- Consults: specify department, name of attending if available, and reason

- Code status: full code/DNR/no vent/no CPR etc.

- Vital: frequency of vitals, special monitors (cardiac, telemetry, continuous O_2 sat)

- Allergies: specify drug, food, or product and type of reaction, NKDA (no known drug allergies)

- Activity: bed rest, BRP (bathroom privilege), ad lib

- Nursing: daily weight, I&O, wound care, dressing changes, bed position

  Call MD parameters: if T > 38°C, BP > 160/90 or < 80/50, O_2 sat < 90%

- Diet: NPO, regular, diabetic, soft diet, clear liquid

- IV fluid: type of fluid and rate, Hep-Lock with q shift flush, TKO (titrate to keep open)

- Meds: specify med, dose, and frequency including prn orders

- Labs: specify name and time of test (STAT, routine, in a.m.)

- Radiology: CXR, CT, MRI, and so on

- Extra: miscellaneous

- Your name and pager number

TABLE 20–2: Progress Note (SOAP Note): Time and Date

- Subjective: a brief summary of how patient feels, any complaints. Psychosocial information, type of procedure and reason why they were performed

- Objective: vital signs, I&O, weights

  Physical examination

  Labs and studies

  Summarize medications

- Assessment: assessment of the patient's complaints and data and draw your conclusions and evaluation of each problem

- Plan: base your plan for the patient's current problems

- Your name and pager number

TABLE 20–3: Procedure Note: Time and Date

- Patient's name and medical record number
- Admission date
- Type of procedure performed
- Date procedure
- Consent
- Pros and cons of the procedure
- Indication of the procedure
- Supervising physician or resident
- Description of the procedure (prep, anesthesia, technique, instruments used, and type of suture used)
- Complication
- Status of patient after procedure
- Your name and pager number

TABLE 20–4: Discharge Note: Time and Date

- Patient's name and medical record number
- Admission date
- Discharge date
- Admission diagnosis
- Discharge diagnosis (can be more than one)
- Admission summary
- Hospital course (brief)
  1. Labs
  2. Consults
  3. Change in therapy
  4. Procedures
- Discharge medications
- Disposition
  1. Place and condition upon discharge
  2. Follow up labs
  3. Follow up appointments
  4. Special instructions
- Your name and pager number

TABLE 20–5: Preoperative Note: Time and Date

- Patient's name and medical record number
- Admission date
- Preoperative diagnosis
- Type of surgery or procedure planned
- Consents
- Physical examination
- Labs and radiologic studies
- ECG findings
- Blood type and type and cross
- Orders (preoperative preparations, e.g., prophylactic antibiotics, skin prep, and NPO)
- Your name and pager number

TABLE 20–6: Operative Note: Time and Date

- Patient's name and medical record number
- Admission date
- Preoperative diagnosis
- Postoperative diagnosis
- Type of surgery or procedure performed
- Date of surgery or procedure
- Attending physician and name of resident or medical student
- Type of anesthesia given
- Findings during surgery or procedure
- Type and amount of fluid infused
- Estimated blood loss (EBL)
- Type and location of drain placed
- Complication during surgery or procedure
- Specimen sent for pathology
- Current condition and disposition
- Your name and pager number

TABLE 20–7: Postoperative Note: Time and Date

• Patient's name and medical record number
• Admission date
• Type of surgery or procedure performed
• Date of surgery or procedure
• Postoperative date and day
• SOAP note
• S: subjective feeling of patient (e.g., any complaints, N/V, pain control, passing gas, and voiding)
• O: 1. Vitals and O_2 saturation
2. Total I/O and urinary output
3. Physical examination
4. Lab
5. Medications and oxygen delivery
• Assessment
• Plan (diet, activity, medications)
• Your name and pager number

TABLE 20–8: Labor and Delivery Note: Time and Date

- Patient's name, medical record number, age, race, gravida, para, and abortion status

- Delivery at gestational age

- Delivery date and time

- Type of delivery: delivery type, time and date

  (If C-section → document reason for C-section)

- Sex of infant and weight, APGAR scores

- Delivered by and assisted by

- Rupture of membrane: spontaneous vs. AROM, time of rupture (date and time)

  - Type of fluid noted after rupture (meconium vs. clear)

- Monitoring during labor: EFM, IFM, or IUPC

- Type of analgesia/anesthesia:

- Medications or fluids given during labor and delivery

- Delivery of placenta: time, actively extracted with gentle traction vs. spontaneous, intact vs. not intact

- Estimated blood loss (EBL)

- Placenta and umbilical cord: document no. of arteries and no. of veins (2 arteries and 1 vein)

  - Document whether cord blood was sent for analysis

- Laceration noted: cervical, vaginal, labial, or rectum, repaired or not

  - If repaired → type of sutures used and type of knots used

(continued)

TABLE 20–8 (Continued)

- Complication during labor and delivery (episiotomy, suction), forceps or vacuum used and reason whether infant was suctioned after delivery or at perineum

- Duration of labor (stage 1, 2, and 3)

- Current patient condition

- Your name and pager number

TABLE 20–9: Postpartum Note: Time and Date

- Patient's name, medical record number, age, race, gravida, para, and abortion status

- Delivery type, time and date

- SOAP note

- S: subjective feeling of patient (e.g., any complaints, pain control, bleeding [frequency and intensity], urination, bowel movement, flatulence, breast or bottle feeding, contraception, and circumcision if male infant)

- O: 1. Vitals

  2. I/O

  3. Physical examination: (uterus should be firm, fundal height, if incision [if applicable] is healing)

  4. Lab (Hg usually performed 12–16 h postpartum)

  5. Medications and oxygen delivery

- Assessment (include PPD no. [postpartum day])

- Plan

- Your name and pager number

TABLE 20–10: Newborn Note: Time and Date

- Newborn's name if available, medical record number and birth weight and height

- Mother's name and age and gravida and para status

- Mother's past medical history

- Home environment and emotional support

- Mother's status in following:

  - Blood type and Rh status

  - Hep B status

  - Rubella status

  - GBS status

  - Syphilis status

  - HIV status

- Gestational age and birth date and time

- Type of delivery and complications during labor and APGAR score

- Vitals

- Physical examination (see Table 14–3)

- Neonate's current weight and head circumference

(continued)

TABLE 20–10 (Continued)

- Feeding (breast vs. bottle [type] and frequency of feeding), voiding frequency and stooling frequency

- LATCH score (score determining how good mother's technique is for breast feeding)

- Circumcision status

- Transcutaneous bilirubin (if > 36 h of age)

- Name of pediatrician and phone number

- Current condition

- Your name and pager number

TABLE 20-11: Death Note: Time and Date

- Patient's name and medical record number

- Admission date

- Today's date

- Time you were notified by a nurse

- Time the patient was seen by you

- Document the following examination being absent:

  1. Respiration (should be absent)

  2. Pulse (should be absent)

  3. Pupillary reaction (should be fixed and dilated)

  4. Reaction to pain stimuli → sternal rub or pressing on nail bed with metal (should be absent)

- Time the patient was pronounced dead, also document the date

- Document probable cause of death

- Document whether the patient's family was notified about having an autopsy performed

- Document that next of kin was notified.

- Inform coroner (If required)

- Document that the family member and primary care physician were notified.

- Your name and pager number

TABLE 20–12: Prescription Writing: Time and Date

- Patient's full name
- Today's date
- Drug name; dosage → metoprolol 50 mg
- Frequency and route → sig: 1 tab PO bid
- Quantity to dispense → # 60 or "QS" (quantity sufficient): number of days, weeks, months
- Number of refill → 2 refills
- Your signature, name, and license number

21
Normal Lab Values and Fluids*

---

*Normal ranges will vary between labs.

TABLE 21–1: IV Fluid Contents/Dextrose							
	IV Fluid Contents					**Dextrose**	
	Na	K	Cl	HCO_3	mOsm/L	g/L	kcal/L
NS	154		154		286		
$^1/_2$ NS	77		77		143		
3% saline	513		513		1026		
5% saline	855		855		1710		
D_5NS	154		154		564	50	170
D_5W					278	50	170
$D_{10}W$					556	100	340
$D_{20}W$					1112	200	680
$D_{50}W$					2780	500	1700
LR	130	4	109	28	272	50	0
D_5RL	130	4	109	28	525	50	170

TABLE 21–2: Hematology

Hgb: ♂ = 13.5–17.5, ♀ = 12–16 g/dL	Platelet: 150–450 × 10^3/mm^3	INR = 2–3
Hct: ♂ = 39–49, ♀ = 35–45%	PT = <12 s	Haptoglobin: 2–140 mg/dL
RBCs: = 4.3–5.7, ♀ = 3.8–5.1 × 10^8 μL	aPTT = <28 s	HbA1C = 5–7%
MCV = 80–100 μm^3	TT = 13–20 s	ESR: ♂ = 0–15 mm/h ♀ = 0–20 mm/h
MCH = 25–35 pg/cell	Bleeding time = 2–7 min	
MCHC = 31–36% Hb/cell	Fibrinogen: 150–350 mg/dL	Plasma volume: ♂ = 25–43 mL/kg ♀ = 28–45 mL/kg
Reticulocyte count: 0.5–1.5% cells	FDP = <10 μg/mL	
Corrected reticulocyte count: (Hct/45) × reticulocyte%	Iron: ♂ = 65–175 μg/dL ♀ = 50–170 μg/dL	Red cell volume: ♂ = 20–36 mL/kg ♀ = 19–31 mL/kg
WBC (leukocyte): 4. 5–11 × 10^3/μL	Ferritin: ♂ = 15–200 ng/mL ♀ = 12–150 ng/mL	
Neutrophil = 57–67%		

(continued)

TABLE 21–2 (Continued)		
Segs = 54–62%	TIBC = 250–400 µg/dL	CD_4 = > 500/mm^3
Bands = 3–5%	Transferrin = 200–400 mg/dL	B_{12} = 100–700 pg/mL
Lymphocytes = 25–33%	Iron sat. = ♂ = 20–50% ♀ = 15–50%	Folate = 3–15 ng/mL
Basophils = 0–0.75%		Pb = <10 µg/dL
Monocytes = 3–7%		
Eosinophils = 1–3%		

TABLE 21–3: Chemistry		
Na^+ = 135–146 meq/L	Anion gap = 7–16 meq/L	Lactate = 0.5–1.66 mmol/L
K^+ = 3.5–5 meq/L	Osmolality = 275–295 mOsmol/kg	Immunoglobulin: IgA = 70–312 mg/dL IgG = 640–1350 mg/dL IgM = 56–350 mg/dL IgE = 0–380 IU/mL
Cl = 95–105 meq/L	Protein: Total (recumbent) = 6–7.8 g/dL Albumin = 3.5–5.5 g/dL Globulin = 2.3–3.5 g/dL	
HCO_3 = 22–28 meq/L		
BUN = 7–18 mg/dL		
Creatinine = 0.6–1.2 mg/dL		
Mg = 1.3–2.4 meq/L	Uric acid = 3–8.2 mg/dL	Creatinine kinase: ♂ = 25–90 U/L ♀ = 10–70 U/L
PO_4 = 2.5–4.5 mg/dL	Zn = 55–135 µg/dL	
Ca^+ = 8.4–10.2 mg/dL, ionized (free) = 4.65–5.28 mg/dL		LDH = 45–90 U/L

TABLE 21–4: Liver Function		
AST (SGOT) = 15–40 U/L	Bilirubin conjugated = 0–0.3 mg/dL	
ALT (SGPT) = 10–40 U/L	Bilirubin total = 0.1–1 mg/dL	
Alk PO_4: ♂ = 30–100 U/L, ♀ = 45–115 U/L	Ammonia = 10–50 μmol/L	
GGT = 0–50 U/L		
Lipase: <130 U/L	Amylase: 0–140 U/dL	C-peptide: 0.70–1.89 ng/mL

TABLE 21–5: Hormones	
Aldosterone Supine = 3–10, upright = 5–30 ng/dL	Progesterone Follicular phase = 0.15–0.7 ng/mL
Cortisol: 8 a.m. = 6–23, 4 p.m. = 3–15 µg/dL,	Luteal phase = 2–25 ng/mL
10 p.m. = <50% of 8 a.m.	Prolactin = <20 ng/mL
Gastrin: <100 pg/mL	PTH: 10–65 pg/mL
Growth hormone ♂ = <2 ng/mL, ♀ = <10 ng/mL	Sperm: 20–200 million/mL
>60 years of age → ♂ = <10 ng/mL ♀ = <14 ng/mL	Testosterone: ♂ (Free) = 52–280 pg/mL
	Total = 300–1000 ng/dL
Estrogen: Follicular phase = 60–200 g/dL	T_3 resin uptake: 25–35%
Luteal phase = 160–400 g/dL	T_3 total: 100–200 ng/dL
Menopause = 130 pg/dL	T_4 total: 5–12 µg/dL
FSH: Follicular phase = 1–9 mU/mL	T_4 free: 0.8–2.3 ng/dL
Ovulation = 6–26 mU/mL	TBG: 16–34 µg/dL

(continued)

TABLE 21–5 (Continued)	
Luteal phase = 1–9 mU/mL	TSH: <10 µU/mL
Menopause = 40–250 mU/mL	>60 years of age: ♂ = 2–7.3 µU/mL
LH: Follicular phase = 1–12 mU/mL	♀ = 2–16.8 µU/mL
Ovulation = 16–104 mU/mL	Radioactive iodide uptake (I^{123}): 10–30%
Luteal phase = 1–12 mU/mL	
Menopause = 30–200 mU/mL	

TABLE 21–6: Fasting Lipid Values			
Total Cholesterol (mg/dL)		**HDL-C (mg/dL)**	
Desirable	<200	Low	<40
Borderline high	200–239	High	>60
High	>240		
LDL-C (mg/dL)		**Triglycerides (mg/dL)**	
Optimal	<100	Normal	150
Above optimal for CHD equivalent	100–129	Borderline	150–199
Borderline high	130–159	High	200–500
High	160–189	Very high	>500
Very high	>190		
Source: NCEP ATP III.			

TABLE 21–7: Blood Gas					
	pH	PCO_2	PO_2	HCO_3	O_2Sat
Arterial	7.35–7.45	35–45	75–100	22–28 meq/L	>95%
Venous	7.32–7.42	41–51	25–40	24–28 meq/L	60–85%

TABLE 21–8: CSF Fluid			
Pressure	WBC	Protein	Glucose
60–18 mmH$_2$O	0–5/μL	15–45 mg/dL	40–80 mg/dL

TABLE 21–9: Synovial Fluid				
WBC	Protein	Glucose	Uric Acid	LDH
<200/μL	<3 g/dL	>50 mg/dL	<8 mg/dL	Less than serum

TABLE 21–10: Urine			
Specific gravity	1.015–1.030	Ca^+	100–300 mg/day
Osmol	600–1400 mOsmol/kg	K^+	25–125 meq/day
Creatinine: ♂	14–26 mg/kg/day	Na^+	40–220 meq/day
♀	11–22 mg/kg/day	PO_4^-	0.4–1.3 g/day
CrClearance[a] ♂	100–150 mL/min	Glucose	<0.5 g/day
♀	90–140 mL/min	Protein	10–100 mg/day
Urea nitrogen	12–20 g/day	Albumin	10–100 mg/day
Uric acid	250–750 mg/day	Amylase	1–17 unit/h

[a]CrClearance varies with BMI (body mass index).

TABLE 21–11: Toxin Levels		
Acetaminophen = >200 µg/mL	Alcohol level (mg/dL) >100 = intoxication	Lead = >100 mg/dL
CO Hgb = >20%	>200 = lethargic	Methanol = >200 mg/L
Ethylene glycol = >20 mg/dL	>300 = coma	Salicylate = 300 µg/mL

TABLE 21–12: Commonly Used Drugs and their Therapeutic Levels			
Medication	**Range**	**Medication**	**Range**
Carbamazepine (Tegretol)	4–12 µg/mL	Phenytoin (Dilantin)	10–20 µg/mL
Digoxin (Lanoxin)	0.8–2.0 ng/mL	Free phenytoin	1–2 µg/mL
Disopyramide (Norpace)	2–5 µg/mL	Procainamide (Pronestyl)	3–10 µg/mL
Doxepin (Sinequan)	75–200 ng/mL	Quinidine (Quinaglute Dura)	1.5–5 µg/mL
Ethosuximide (Zarontin)	40–100 µg/mL		
Flecainide (Tambocor)	0.2–1 µg/mL	Theophylline (Theo-Dur)	10–20 µg/mL
Imipramine (Tofranil)	150–300 µg/mL	Tobramycin (TobraDex)	4–6 µg/mL
Lidocaine (Xylocaine)	1.5–6 µg/mL	Tocainide (Tonocard)	4–10 µg/mL
Lithium (Lithobid)	0.6–1.2 meq/L	Valproic acid (Depakote)	
Phenobarbital (Luminal)	10–40 µg/mL	→ Acute mania	50–125 µg/mL
		→ Epilepsy	50–100 µg/mL

(continued)

TABLE 21–12 (Continued)

Note

- The therapeutic range of some drugs may vary depending on the reference lab used.

- Correct phenytoin (Dilantin) level for low albumin or check free dilantin level.

- Correct phenytoin (Dilantin) for low albumin = measured Dilantin (albumin × 0.2) + 0.1.

- Correct phenytoin (Dilantin) in renal failure = measured Dilantin (albumin × 0.1) + 0.1.

- Phenytoin has a narrow therapeutic range, necessitating the monitoring of serum levels. It is highly protein bound to albumin and only the free fraction of the drug is active.

- Monitor free serum phenytoin levels and a baseline albumin level due to the potential for increased phenytoin levels and toxicity in the following conditions:

  1. Renal failure (CrCl less than 25 mL/min): phenytoin binding is altered due to ↓ affinity of plasma proteins.

  2. Hypoalbuminemia (<3.5 g/dL): may result in an increased free fraction of phenytoin.

  3. Hepatic disease: results in decreased metabolism of phenytoin.

TABLE 21–13: Normal Lab in Pregnancy		
Lab	**Value**	**Change from Nonpregnant ♀**
WBC	$5–15 \times 10^3/mm^3$	↑
Hgb	11–14 g/dL	↓
Hct	33–42%	↓
Creatinine	<1 mg/dL	↓
BUN	4–12 mg/dL	↓
TSH	0.2–3.5 µU/mL	↓
T_4	7.8–16.2 µg/dL	↑
Thyroid binding globulin (TBG)	19–68 µg/dL	↑
T_3 resin uptake	18–25%	↓
Fibrinogen	400–500 mg/dL	↑
Arterial pH	7.4–7.45	↑
PCO_2	27–32 mmHg	↓
HCO_3	19–25 meq/L	↓

22
Troubleshooting

TABLE 22–1: CMP and CBC Troubleshooting

- Corrected sodium for glucose → Δglucose 100 = $1.6 - 2$ Na^+ (meq)

- Corrected sodium for triglyceride → Na^+ (meq) = plasma TG (g/L) $\times$ 0.002

- Corrected sodium for plasma protein → Na^+ (meq) = plasma protein $-$ 8 (g/dL) $\times$ 0.025

- ΔCO_2 of 10 mmHg acute = ΔpH 0.8 = ΔHCO_3 of 5 meq/L

- ΔCO_2 of 10 mmHg chronic = ΔpH 0.3

- Corrected calcium and anion gap Δalbumin 1 g = ΔCa 0.8, anion gap 2.2

↑ WBC		
• Acute infection	• Acute/chronic inflammatory disease	
• Stress induced	• Tissue necrosis (burn, MI, neoplasia)	
• Small bowel obstruction	• Collagen vascular disease	
• Thyroid storm	**Drug induced**	
• DKA	• ACE (eosinophils)	• Heparin
• Trauma (internal or external)	• Bactrim	• Histamines
• Leukemia	• Digitalis	• Lithium
• Hypoadrenalism	• Epinephrine	• Steroids

TABLE 22–1 (Continued)	
↑ **H&H**	↓ **H&H**
• Cigarette smoking	• Blood loss
• COPD	• Pregnancy
• Hemoconcentration (shock, surgery, burn, dehydration)	• Hemodilution
• Polycythemia	• Edematous state
• High altitude	
↑ **BUN**	↓ **BUN**
• Prerenal azotemia	• Chronic ETOH ingestion (liver disease)
• Renal disease	• SIADH
• Postrenal disease	• Malnutrition
• GI bleed	• Pregnancy
• Steroids	• Over hydration
↑ **Liver Enzymes**	
↑ **AST (Acute)**	
• Liver disease/damage	• Shock
• Hemolysis	• Acute pancreatitis
• Cholestasis	• Burn (3rd degree)
• MI or myocarditis	• Seizure
• Skeletal muscle disease	• Heparin therapy

(continued)

TABLE 22–1 (Continued)

↑ ALT

• Liver disease/damage	• Disease of muscle metabolism
• Celiac sprue	• Strenuous exercise

Medication Associated with ↑ AST and ↑ ALT

• PCN (synthetic)	• NSAIDs
• Ciprofloxacin	• Glipizide
• Nitrofurantoin	• Heparin
• Ketoconazole, fluconazole	• Steroids
• Statins	• Cocaine, NMDA, PCP, glues, solvents

↑ Alkaline Phosphatase

• Intra- and extrahepatic liver damage	• Bone disease (osteoblastic)
• Congestive heart failure (CHF)	• 2° Hyperparathyroidism
• Acute pancreatitis	• Renal disease
• Infectious mononucleosis	• Malabsorption
• CMV	• Pregnancy
• Sepsis	• Sarcoidosis
• Perforation of bowel	• Amyloidosis

TABLE 22–1 (Continued)	
Check Before Ordering the Following:	**Check After Ordering the Following:**
• BP → nitroglycerin, cough syrup	• Topamax → HCO_3
• Bun/Cr → ACE	• Coumadin → INR/PT
→ Spiral CT/other contrast studies	• HCTZ → K^+
→ Bisphosphonates	• Metformin → lactic acid, BUN/Cr
→ NSAID	• Nitroprusside → thiocyanate level
→ Lantus insulin	• Heparin → PTT, platelet
→ Bactrim	• Trileptal → Na^+
• LFT → statin, Dilantin	
• CBC → carbamazepine	
• Stool guaiac → Heparin/anticoagulants/ warfarin	

TABLE 22–2: Drug-induced Conditions

- ACE → ↑ K^+ and ↑ eosinophils

- Depakote → hyponatremia

- Heparin/H_2 blockers → ↓ platelet

- Metformin → lactic acidosis

- NSAID → ↑ K^+

- Oxytocin → ↓ Na^+

- Reglan → ↓ BP

- Seroquel → ↓ Na^+

- Steroids → ↑ glucose, Na^+, WBC, BP, BUN

  → ↓ K^+, calcium, platelet

- Topamax → hyperchloremic metabolic alkalosis

TABLE 22–3: Important Drug–Drug Interaction

- Anticoagulants (warfarin, anisindione, dicumarol) ↔ thyroid hormone

- Allopurinol ↔ thiopurines (azathioprine and mercaptopurine)

- Benzodiazepines ↔ azole antifungal (fluconazole, itraconazole, and ketoconazole)

- Carbamazepine ↔ propoxyphene

- Cyclosporine ↔ rifamycins (rifampin, rifabutin, and rifapentine)

- Dextromethorphan ↔ MAOI (isocarboxazid, phenelzine, selegiline, and tranylcypromine)

- Digoxin ↔ clarithromycin

- Ergot alkaloids (ergotamine, methysergide, dihydroergotamine) ↔ macrolides (clarithromycin, erythromycin, and troleandomycin)

- Estrogen–progestin products (OCP) ↔ rifampin

- Ganciclovir ↔ zidovudine

- HCTZ ↔ lithium

- MAOI ↔ amphetamines, diethylpropion, Demerol, dopamine, ephedrine, isometheptene mucate, mazindol, metaraminol, phenylephrine, pseudoephedrine, and SSRI

- Meperidine (Demerol) ↔ MAOI

- Methotrexate ↔ trimethoprim

- Nitrates ↔ sildenafil

(continued)

TABLE 22–3 (Continued)

- Pimozide ↔ macrolides (clarithromycin, dirithromycin, erythromycin, and troleandomycin)

- Azole antifungal
  (fluconazole, itraconazole, and ketoconazole)

- SSRI ↔ MAOI

- Theophylline ↔ quinolone (ciprofloxacin and enoxacin), fluvoxamine

- Warfarin ↔ Gingko biloba

- Warfarin ↔ barbiturates, cimetidine, fibric acid derivatives (Clofibrate, fenofibrate, gemfibrozil), NSAIDs, and sulfinpyrazone

Reprinted with permission: Malone DC, Abarca J, Hansten PD, et al. Medications likely to be dispensed in community pharmacy. *J Am Pharm Assoc.* 2004; 44:142–151.

TABLE 22–4: Drug and Important Properties

- ACE: when placing patient on ACE, start them on a shorter-acting ACE due to its side effect of angioedema (ACE ↑ release of bradykinin)

- Calcium channel blocker: edema

- Dig toxicity ↑ by → hypocalcemia and hypokalemia

- Effexor: ↑ BP

- Heparin/Depo-Provera: can cause osteoporosis

- Mefloquine: psychosis

- Metformin: avoid in renal insufficiency (Cr > 3), also avoid prior to IV contrast use and 48 h after IV contrast use

- NSAIDs: avoid in renal insufficiency

- Paxil: can cause flu like symptoms

- Steroids: can cause osteoporosis, psychosis

- TCA: cardiac arrhythmia

- Demerol/selegiline/dextromethorphan: can cause serotonin syndrome

- Wellbutrin can be used for smoking cessation, can decrease threshold for seizure

TABLE 22–5: Steroid Equivalent Dosing

Steroid	Equivalent Dose
• Dexamethasone (Decadron, Dexon, and Hexadrol)	0.75 mg
Tablet: 0.25, 0.5, 0.75, 1, 1.5, 2, 4 mg	
Elixir: 0.5 mg/5 mL, injection: 4 mg/mL, Intensol: 1 mg/mL	
• Methylprednisolone (Medrol, Solu-Medrol, Depo-Medrol)	4 mg
Tablet: 2, 4, 16, 24 mg	
Injection: 40, 125, 500 mg, 1 g	
Injection suspension: 80 mg/mL	
• Prednisolone (Delta-Cortef, Prelone syrup, Prediapred)	5 mg
Tablet: 5 mg	
Liquid: 5 mg/5 mL	
Syrup: 15 mg/5 mL	

TABLE 22–5 (Continued)	
• Prednisone (Deltasone, Liquid pred, Orasone)	5 mg
Tablet: 1, 2.5, 5, 10, 20, 50 mg	
Liquid: 5 mg/5 mL	
• Hydrocortisone (Cortef)	20 mg
Tablet: 5, 10, 20 mg	
Suspension: 10 mg/5 mL	
Injection: 50 mg/mL	
• Cortisone (Cortone)	25 mg
Tablet: 5 mg	
Injection: 50 mg/mL	

TABLE 22–6: Radiologic Test Precautions

- Check BUN/Cr before ordering spiral CT, if high consider alternative test or premedication with *N*-acetylcysteine

- When looking for an abscess or osteomyelitis and is unable to fit into a CT/MRI scan

  → Use WBC scan (Indium scan) to find the source of infection

TABLE 22–7: MRI Contraindications

• Cardiac pacemaker	• Implanted cardiac defibrillator
• Aneurysm clips	• Carotid artery vascular clamp
• Neurostimulator	• Implanted drug infusion device
• Bone growth/fusion stimulator	• Cochlear, otologic, or ear implant
• Metallic splinters in eye	• Hemostatic CNS clips

TABLE 22–8: Useful Web sites	
www.accessmedicine.com	Medical info (*Harrison's Online*, Lange Currents and *CMDT*)
www.acponline.org	*The American College of Physicians*
www.ACC.org	*The American College of Cardiology*
www.ama-assn.org	*The American Medical Association*
www.bmj.com	*The British Medical Journal*
www.cdc.gov	The Center of Disease Control and Prevention
http://Dermis.multimedica.de	Dermatology atlas and info
www.Diabetes.org	*The American Diabetes Association*
www.EMedicine.com	Medical info
www.EmedHome.com	Emergency Medicine info

(continued)

TABLE 22–5 (Continued)	
www.aaem.org	*American Academy of Emergency Medicine*
www.ems-c.org	Emergency Medical Services for Children
www.FamilyMedicine.Medscape.com	Medical info
www.FamilyPracticeNotebook.com	Medical info
www.FDA.gov	The Food and Drug Administration
www.FreeBooks4Doctors.com	Online books
www.Guidelines.gov	Guidelines and recommendations
www.Harrisonsonline.com	*Harrison's Online*
www.Healthfinder.gov	Medical info
www.Immunize.org	Immunization update
www.MDConsult.com	Medical info
www.MedicalConferences. com	Medical Conferences
www.medlineplus.gov	The National Library of Medicine
www.Medscape.com	Medicine search site and Medical library

TABLE 22–5 (Continued)	
www.Merck.com/pubs/mmanual	Medical info
www.Merck.com/pubs/mm_geriatrics	Medical info
www.merckmedicus.com	Medical info
www.Nejm.org	*The New England Journal of Medicine*
www.NIH.gov	The National Institutes of Health
www.postgradmed.com	Medical info
www.vh.org	The Virtual Hospital (Medical info)

23
Common Abbreviations

TABLE 23–1: Common Abbreviations
A
a—arterial
ā —before
Aa—alveolar/arterial
AAA—abdominal aortic aneurysm
AAO × 3—awake, alert, oriented × 3
abd—abdomen
ABG—arterial blood gas
Ac—before meal
ACLS—advance cardiac life support
Ad lib—as needed/as desired
ADAT—advance diet as tolerated
adm—admission
AF—atrial fibrillation
AFB—acid-fast bacilli
AFP—alpha fetoprotein
AG—anion gap
AKA—above the knee amputation
Alb—albumin
AMA—against medical advice
AMI—acute myocardial infarction
Amp—ampule

TABLE 23–1 (Continued)

ANA—antinuclear antibody

ANCA—antinuclear cytoplasmic antibody

ant—anterior

ante—before

Anti-SMA—antismooth muscle antibody

AP—anteroposterior

Aq—aqueous

AR—aortic regurgitation

ARC—aids-related complex

ARDS—acute respiratory distress syndrome

ARF—acute renal failure

asa—aspirin

ASHD—atherosclerotic heart disease

ASO—antistreptolysin O

ATN—acute tubular necrosis

AVM—arteriovenous malformation

Ax—axillary

AXR—abdominal x-ray

(continued)

TABLE 23–1 (Continued)

B

BBB—bundle branch block

BCx—blood culture

BCP—birth control pill

BE—barium enema

bid—twice a day

BILAT—bilaterally

BILI—bilirubin

BKA—below the knee amputation

BM—bowel movement

BMP—basic metabolic panel

BP—blood pressure

BRBPR—bright red blood per rectum

BRP—bathroom privileges

BSO—bilateral salpingo-oophorectomy

BTL—bilateral tubal ligation

BUN—blood urea nitrogen

BW—body weight

Bx—biopsy

TABLE 23–1 (Continued)
C
c̄ —with
c/o—complains of
C/S—culture and sensitivity
C/sec—cesarean section
Ca—cancer
CABG—coronary artery bypass grafting
CAD—coronary artery disease
cal—calories
cap—capsule
CBC—complete blood count
CBD—common bile duct
CrCl—creatinine clearance
CD—continuous drainage
CHD—coronary heart disease
CHF—congestive heart failure
CK—creatinine kinase
COPD—chronic obstructive pulmonary disease
CPAP—continuous positive airway pressure
CPK—creatine phosphokinase
CPR—cardiopulmonary resuscitation
CPT—chest physiotherapy

(continued)

TABLE 23–1 (Continued)
Cr—creatinine
CRF—chronic renal failure
CSF—cerebrospinal fluid
CTA—clear to auscultation
CTS—carpal tunnel syndrome
CTX—contraction
CV—cardiovascular
CVP—central venous pressure
Cx—culture
CXR—chest x-ray
D
D&C—dilation and curettage
d/c—discontinue/discharge
D_5W—5% dextrose in water
DAT—diet as tolerated
DBILI—direct bilirubin
DBP—diastolic blood pressure
DDAVP—desmopressin
Decub—decubitus
DI—diabetes insipidus
DIC—disseminated intravascular coagulation
DIP—distal interphalangeal

TABLE 23–1 (Continued)
DJD—degenerative joint disease
DKA—diabetes ketoacidosis
DM—diabetes mellitus
DNR—do not resuscitate
DOA—dead on arrival/date of admission
DOD—date of discharge
DOE—dyspnea on exertion
DPI—dry powder inhaler
DSD—dry sterile dressing
DTR—deep tendon reflexes
DUB—dysfunctional uterine bleeding
DVT—deep vein thrombosis
Dx—diagnosis
dz—disease
E
EBL—estimated blood loss
EBV—Epstein–Barr virus
ECF—extracellular fluid
ECT—electroconvulsive therapy
EDC—estimated date of confinement
EDTA—ethylene diamine tetraacetate
EEG—electroencephalogram

(continued)

TABLE 23–1 (Continued)

EENT—eyes, ears, nose, and throat
EF—ejection fraction
elem—Elemental
EMG—electromyogram
EOMI—extraocular movements intact
EPO—erythropoietin
ERCP—endoscopic retrograde cholangiopancreatography
ESR—erythrocyte sedimentation rate
ET—endotracheal
F
f/u—follow up
FBS—fasting blood sugar
FEN—fluids, electrolytes, nutrition
FEV—forced expiratory volume
FFP—fresh frozen plasma
FHR—fetal heart rate
FHT—fundal height
fl—fluid
FNA—fine needle aspiration
FSH—follicle-stimulating hormone
FUO—fever of unknown origin
FVC—forced vital capacity
fx—fracture

TABLE 23–1 (Continued)
G
GB—gall bladder
Gc—gonococcus
GERD—gastroesophageal reflux disease
GFR—glomerular filtration rate
GSW—gun shot wound
gt/gtt—drop/drops
GVHD—graft versus host disease
H
h/o—history of
HA—headache
Hct—hematocrit
HD—hemodialysis/hospital day
HEENT—head, eyes, ears, nose, and throat
Hgb—hemoglobin
HHA—home health aid
HORF—high output renal failure
HPV—human papilloma virus
hs—bed time (hours of time)
HSM—hepatosplenomegaly
HSV—herpes simplex virus
HTN—hypertension
Hx—history

(continued)

TABLE 23–1 (Continued)
I
I&D—incision and drainage
I&O—intake and output
IABP—intraaortic balloon pump
IBD—inflammatory bowel disease
IBS—irritable bowel syndrome
ICP—intracranial pressure
IDDM—insulin-dependent diabetes mellitus
IM—intramuscular
inj—injection
INR—International normalized ratio
IOP—intraocular pressure
IPPB—intermittent positive pressure breathing
ITP—idiopathic thrombocytopenic purpura
IUD—intrauterine device
IVF—intravenous fluids
IVP—intravenous pyelogram
J
JVD—jugular venous distension
JVP—jugular venous pressure

TABLE 23–1 (Continued)

K

KCl—potassium chloride

KUB—kidney, ureter, and bladder

KVO—keep vein open

L

lac—laceration

LAD—left axis deviation

LAP—laparotomy

lat—lateral

LBBB—left bundle branch block

LBP—lower back pain

LDH—lactate dehydrogenase

LE—lower extremities

LFT—liver function test

LLQ—left lower quadrant

LOC—level of consciousness

LP—lumbar puncture

LUL—left upper lobe

LUQ—left upper quadrant

LVH—left ventricular hypertrophy

(continued)

TABLE 23–1 (Continued)
M
MAP—mean arterial pressure
MAT—multi-focal atrial tachycardia
MCA—middle cerebral artery
MCP—metacarpophalangeal joint
MDI—metered dose inhaler
MIC—minimum inhibitory concentration
MMSE—mini-mental status examination
MODS—multiple organ dysfunction syndrome
MOM—milk of magnesia
MRSA—methicillin resistant staph aureus
MVI—multivitamins
N
N/V—nausea/vomiting
N/V/D—nausea/vomiting/diarrhea
NAD—no acute distress
NB—newborn
NC/AT—normocephalic/atraumatic
NG—nasogastric
NKA—no known allergies
NKDA—no known drug allergies
NPO—nothing by mouth

TABLE 23–1 (Continued)
NPH—normopressure hydrocephalus
NS—normal saline
NSR—normal sinus rhythm
NTG—nitroglycerin
O
OA—oral airway
OBS—organic brain syndrome
OD—right eye/overdose
OOB—out of bed
OPD—outpatient department
OS—left eye
Osm—osmolality
OT—occupational therapy
OU—both eyes
P
p̄—after
PA—posterior–anterior
PACU—postanesthesia care unit
pc—after meal
pcr—through
PCWP—pulmonary capillary wedge pressure
PE—pulmonary embolism

(continued)

TABLE 23–1 (Continued)
PERRLA—pupils equal round and reactive to light and accommodation
PFT—pulmonary function test
PID— pelvic inflammatory disease
PIV—peripheral IV
PMD—primary medical doctor
PMI—point of maximum impulse
PND—paroxysmal nocturnal dyspnea
po/PO—by mouth
POD—postoperative day
PR—per rectum
PRBCs—packed red blood cells
prn/PRN—as needed
PROM—premature rupture of membrane
PSA—prostate specific antigen
PSGN—poststreptococcal glomerulonephritis
PSVT—paroxysmal supraventricular tachycardia
PTA—prior to admission
PTX—pneumothorax
PUD—peptic ulcer disease
PWP—pulmonary wedge pressure
Px—prognosis

TABLE 23–1 (Continued)
Q
q—every
q2h—every two hour
qd—every day, Daily
qh—every night or bedtime
qhs—every night
qid—four times a day
qod—every other day
qs—quantity sufficient
R
RR—respiratory rate
R/O—rule out
R/T—related to
RBBB—right bundle branch block
RDW—red cell distribution width
RF—rheumatoid factor
RLL—right lower lobe
RLQ—right lower quadrant
RML—right middle lobe
ROM—range of motion
ROS—review of system
RPGN—rapidly progressive glomerular nephritis

(continued)

TABLE 23–1 (Continued)
RPR—rapid plasma reagin
RRR—regular rate and rhythm
RSR—regular sinus rhythm
RTA—renal tubular acidosis
RTC—return to clinic
RTO—return to office
RUL— right upper lobe
RUQ—right upper quadrant
RVH—renovascular hypertension
—right ventricular hypertrophy
RXN—reaction
S
$\bar{s}$—without
S/NT/ND—soft/nontender/nondistended
S/P—status post
SAH—subarachnoid hemorrhage
SBE—subacute bacterial endocarditis
SBFT—small bowel follow through
SBP—spontaneous bacterial peritonitis/systolic BP
SGA—small for gestational age
SIADH—syndrome of inappropriate ADH
Sig—direction

TABLE 23–1 (Continued)
SL—sublingual
SOB—shortness of breath
SOC—state of consciousness
sol—solution
SOM—serous otitis media
SPA—salt poor albumin
SC/Sub Q—subcutaneous
ss—half
SSE—soap solution enema
SSS—sick sinus syndrome
SVC—superior vena cava
SVT—supraventricular tachycardia
Sx—symptom
Sz—seizure
T
T&A—tonsillectomy and adenoidectomy
T/C—throat culture
tab—tablet
TAH—total abdominal hysterectomy
Tbs—table spoon
TBW—total body water
TENS—transcutaneous electric nerve stimulation

(continued)

TABLE 23–1 (Continued)
TIA—transient ischemic attack
tid—three times a day
TIPS—transjugular intrahepatic portosystemic shunt
TKO—to keep open
TLC—total lung capacity
TM—tympanic membrane
TO—telephone order
TOLAC—trial of labor after cesarean
TPN—total parenteral nutrition
Tsp—teaspoon
TURP—transurethral resection of prostate
Tx—treatment/therapy
U
U/S—ultrasound
UA—urine analysis
UCx—urine culture
UE—upper extremity
UGI—upper GI
ung—ointment
URI—upper respiratory infection
Ut Dict—as directed
UTI—urinary tract infection

TABLE 23–1 (Continued)

V

VBAC—vaginal birth after cesarean

VCUG—voiding cystourethrogram

VDRL—venereal disease research lab

VO—verbal order

VS—vital signs

VSD—ventricular septal defect

W

WBAT—weight bearing as tolerated

WBC—white blood cell

WNL—within normal limit

wt—weight

X

×—times/multiply

XRT—radiation therapy

Y

y/o—years old

Z

z—dram

Voleenia

FIGURE 24-1: Near Vision Testing

E	O	P	Z	T	L	160 in.
T	D	P	C	F	Z	80 in.
D	Z	E	L	C	F	56 in.
F	E	P	C	T	L	48 in.
P	T	L	F	C	Z	40 in.
E	L	Z	T	C	O	32 in.
D	Z	E	L	P	T	24 in.
L	O	P	F	Z	E	20 in.
E	L	T	C	P	P	16 in.

Hold at 16 in.

FIGURE 24-2: Pupil Size (mm)

Pupil size (mm)

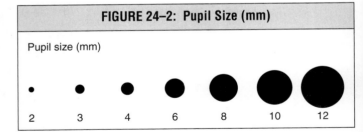

2   3   4   6   8   10   12

Index

Page numbers followed by *f* refer to figures.